Design of a Retainable Keratoprosthesis: History, Design, and Evaluation in Cats

John C. Barber, MD

AuthorHouse™
1663 Liberty Drive
Bloomington, IN 47403
www.authorhouse.com
Phone: 1-800-839-8640

First published by AuthorHouse   03/14/2011

ISBN: 978-1-4567-3130-4 (sc)

Library of Congress Control Number: 2011902356

Printed in the United States of America

This book is printed on acid-free paper.

To the eight million people, worldwide, who could have vision restored by a retainable keratoprosthesis

CONTENTS

Part One   **Executive Summary**   1
Purpose
Method
Results
Conclusions

Part Two   **Introduction**   3

Part Three   **History of Keratoprostheses**   5

The early history of keratoprostheses
Evaluation of prosthesis design styles

Part Four   **Causes of Prosthesis Failure**   13
Mechanical causes of prosthesis failure
Biological causes of prosthesis failure

Part Five   **Design Solutions for Prosthesis Problems**   19

Prosthesis core
Prosthesis flange or skirt

Part Six   **Psychological Considerations**   25

Part Seven   **Current Prostheses**   27

Osteo-odono-keratoprosthesis
Worst Champagne cork prosthesis and Singh prosthesis
Dohlman type II prosthesis
Seoul prosthesis
Legeais prosthesis
Chirila prosthesis
Caldwell prosthesis

Part Eight   **Design of a New Prosthesis**   29
Core
Skirt

Part Nine   **Animal Research**   31
Materials and methods
Experimental animals
Experimental procedures
Evaluation procedures
Results
Discussion

Acknowledgments   43
References   44

ILLUSTRATIONS

1. Schematic drawings of keratoprosthesis design types   8
2. Keratoprosthesis of a new composite design   30
3. Frontal view of the right eye of a cat with prosthesis, six months   36
4. Same eye as in figure 3, lateral view, six months   36
5. Frontal view of cat with keratoprosthesis in right eye.   37
6. Section of cat eye with prosthesis in place, end of study   38
7. Section of cornea containing the Proplast® skirt material (X50)   39
8. Section of cornea containing the Proplast® skirt material (X125)   39

TABLES

Table1. Ratios of Forces on the Prosthesis to Supporting Areas
of the Cornea, Based on Radius of the Core   15

Part One

Summary

Purpose This book will review the history of keratoprostheses to be able to learn which design features enhance prosthesis retention and function. It will also explain the design and testing of a keratoprosthesis that incorporates these design features. The new prosthesis design contains features that have been shown to enhance the function and retention of prostheses. The animal study was designed to determine whether that prosthesis will be retained for a significant length of time in the cat cornea to justify the use of the new prosthesis in human patients.

Method The history of Keratoprostheses was reviewed extensively. The best features of prior keratoprostheses were incorporated into the design of a new prosthesis. Keratoprostheses, made with polymethyl methacrylamide (PMMA) cores and Proplast® skirts, were implanted into intralamellar pockets in the cornea of one eye each of ten American short hair cats in a prospective, non blinded study. The study was conducted in the Department of Ophthalmology of the University of Texas Medical Branch. The cats were examined for the duration of prosthesis retention (to a maximum of six months), and for occurrence of complications including flap retraction or overgrowth, loss of stability, infection, retroprosthetic membranes, retinal detachment, and glaucoma. At the end of the study, all eyes were examined histologically for evidence of fibrovascular implant stabilization, epithelial downgrowth, retroprosthetic membranes, retinal detachment, and intraocular inflammation.

Results Nine out of ten prostheses were retained for the full six months. On histological examination all nine showed total incorporation of the skirt material. Two eyes developed retraction of the covering conjunctival flap, which was surgically corrected. The only other complication was retroprosthetic membrane formation in two eyes—one in the eye from which the prosthesis was extruded.

Conclusions A keratoprosthesis with an anterior overhanging flange, well-bonded core and skirt, posterior core of conical shape, and skirt material with good biointegration potential can be retained in the cat cornea without major complications for at least six months. This prosthesis is now ready for human trials in patients that are not suitable for conventional corneal transplants.

Part Two

Introduction

The cornea is the clear window which allows light to enter the eye. The clarity and shape of that window determine the quality of vision. Both the clarity and shape can be altered by diseases which affect the cornea. Corneal diseases that scar or cloud the cornea have been among the leading causes of blindness through out the world for centuries. Long before the first tissue corneal transplant was attempted, corneal blindness caused physicians to consider placing transparent materials into the cornea to maintain a clear pathway for light to enter the eye. Many unsuccessful attempts were made to place materials into the cornea.

Grafting of the human cornea was first done successfully in 1904 by Zirm. It is ironic that this first successful human keratoplasty was done in a patient who had received a severe chemical burn of the eye. A successful corneal transplant in an eye which has been chemically burned is an achievement that remains difficult to repeat today.

Great strides have been made in maintaining the clarity of corneal transplants. However, for certain diseases, transplantation has a very low success rate with high complication and failure rates. Keratoplasty works relatively well as a treatment for primary corneal edema, traumatic scaring, pseudophakic corneal edema, (after cataract extraction with intraocular lens implant), and corneal dystrophy. The success rate continues to be low for grafts to treat alkali burns, ocular cicatricial pemphigoid, Stevens-Johnson syndrome, recurrent herpetic keratitis, and in most patients with decreased tear function. Eyelid distortion and malfunction are also major causes of repeated graft failure.

Religious beliefs and superstitions are major factors in obtaining donor tissue for keratoplasty throughout much of the world, causing a shortage of corneal tissue. An artificial cornea that would not be immunologically rejected, regardless of the reason for keratoplasty, and that could be readily available in all parts of the world would play an important role in restoring vision for millions of people who suffer from corneal blindness. A recent WHO publication puts the number of people worldwide who suffer from blindness from corneal diseases at eight million.

Since first working with Dr. Dohlman in 1971 to 1973, when he was using his early designs, I have devoted over thirty years to the study of keratoprostheses. In the process, I have reviewed the history of keratoprostheses, from the early attempts to the ones currently in use, to determine which design factors contribute to retention of a prosthesis and which ones seem to be detrimental, or do not contribute to the success of a prosthesis.

Most of the current prostheses rely on some form of biointegration, that is the extensive tissue growth into the prosthesis, to stabilize and retain the prosthesis. Facilitation of this biointegration is an important part of a new prosthesis design. Much of the authors research has dealt with the promotion of biointegration and the factors which enhance or inhibit this integration and the biochemistry of corneal melting that occurs at the prosthesis to tissue interface.

All of these factors will be explained in detail in this presentation. The flaws of existing prostheses will be enumerated and explained, along with design improvements intended to correct the design flaws and enhance the retention of a prosthesis of this novel design, created from the best features of prior and existing implants. The author has also developed additional steps and procedures to aid the successful prosthesis integration and retention. These will be detailed in this monograph.

This report also incorporates the animal study in cats that was used to test this new design to determine whether this design is suitable for good tissue incorporation. It will also demonstrate that there is long enough retention of this prosthesis to justify its use in human subjects with corneal blindness.

The author also discusses the ethical problems posed by the use of what has become a short term remedy for a long term problem. Review of prior reports shows that these questions have not been explored or written about by most prosthesis surgeons.

Part Three

History of Keratoprostheses

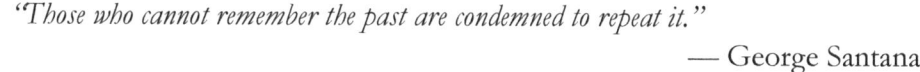

"Those who cannot remember the past are condemned to repeat it."

— George Santana

A brief review is necessary to understand the many designs, materials and surgical approaches which have been tried and the multiple factors which contribute to the success or failure of the past and present keratoprostheses. Once these are understood, a prostheses may be designed that could be retained within the eye for a reasonable period of time to ethically justify use of this prosthesis in the treatment of corneal blindness.

The early history of keratoprostheses The idea of placing a small glass plate into the cornea to create a permanent optical window was originally attributed to Pellier di Quengsy[1]. In 1771, he described a glass lens, surrounded by a highly polished silver ring containing a groove to hold the prosthesis. This ring could be fitted within the scleral rim that remained after the entire cornea was removed. It is not clear from de Quengsy's report whether he actually implanted this device, or was only presenting the idea. His report includes detailed drawings of the device and of the instruments used to implant and maintain it. The report also gives detailed instructions for post operative care and the management of complications.

Actual prosthesis implantations were reported in 1856 by Nussbaum[1,] who used a quartz crystal, and in 1859 by Heusser[2], who used glass. Both implants were retained in the corneas for only a short period of time, which may account for an interval of more than 30 years until the next report of implanting such a device.

In 1891, Dimmer[3] reported two cases in which he had used clear celluloid plates to hold a glass lens in the cornea. This device also lasted for only a short time, being extruded by suppuration (probably infection). About the same time, Salzer[1] performed experiments in which he used egg membranes to hold the lenses in the corneas of rabbits, with only limited success.

There was a hiatus of 60 years until the next report, by Gyorffy[4], who in 1951, described implantation of an acrylic prosthesis in one patient. This was followed by three reports in 1955. Dorzee[5], a Belgian ophthalmologist, published a report of successful use of a spool-shaped keratoprosthesis. The posterior flange was larger than the anterior flange and contained grooves for intentional leakage of aqueous humor to relieve intraocular pressure. He reported that his patient had corrected vision of 0.7 (20/30) five months after implantation.

Also in 1955, Stone[6] reported placing a "highly purified" intralamellar plastic disc at mid depth in the cornea to close a hole through the cornea. Stone did laboratory work on this device, but did not publish further human cases.

Joaquin Barraquer[7] reported use, in a patient in Spain, of the same prosthesis that Dorzee used in the same year, 1955. This patient reportedly had good vision with the prosthesis for five years until necrosis and fistulization caused extrusion of the implant. Barraquer modified this prosthesis by enlarging the posterior plate. This proved to be a mistake, however, as it lead to extrusion in all cases between twenty days and six months after implantation. He then reduced both the size of the posterior plate and the weight of the implant. These changes improved results for some patients, but the extrusion rate remained high.

In 1956, Binder and Binder[8] reported use of a prosthesis made of Plexiglas. Their short term results were favorable, but were followed by later infection and extrusion.

In the 1960's, several research projects were conducted with the goal of producing a workable alloplastic cornea. In search of the ideal alloplastic material, Cardona[9] studied 160 different polymers of acrylic resin. He found them "too toxic" to the cornea and blamed extrusion of the previous implants on their "toxicity". He concluded that all polymers used in the eye must be totally polymerized using ultraviolet light to avoid any leaching of residual monomer, which is very toxic to the eye. At about the same time Choice[10], in England, recommended the use of the material Perspex CQ for prostheses because of success with that material in intraocular lenses. Perspex CQ is an acrylic polymer that is very hard because it is totally polymerized by ultraviolet radiation, making it inert within the eye. Hadley had used Perspex CQ for the first successful intraocular lenses several years before.

In the history of keratoprostheses, many materials have been used for the optical portion including glass, celluloid, Plexiglas, crystal, various types of acrylate, silicone, polycarbonate, hydrogel, urethane, and egg membranes. Today, only glass, polycarbonate, Chirila's hydrogel, urethane, and intraocular quality poly methyl methacrylate (PMMA, a material similar to Perspex CQ), remain in use for the cores.

Evolution of Design Features

Several types of keratoprostheses have been developed and implanted in the past 60 years. These designs need to be evaluated for their affect on the stable retention of the prosthesis in the cornea; the prevention of the growth of conjunctiva over the clear portion (core) of the prosthesis or growth of any epithelium into the eye; the inhibition of retroprosthetic membrane development; and the avoidance of complications such as foreign body reaction, infection, glaucoma, enzymatic erosion.

Cardona[2], developed a so-called "nut and bolt" prosthesis, which included a small, round, acrylic intralamellar plate, the nut, is placed at mid-depth in the corneal stroma (Figure 1, A). A central hole in this plate was threaded to allow the small threaded cylinder to be screwed into the plate through a hole in the cornea. This was replaced by a longer, threaded optical core, the bolt, in a second procedure. This optical core did protrude above the corneal surface to discourage growth of the conjunctiva over the core. If the core extended too far above the cornea, the eyelid would hit it causing problems.

Keratoprosthesis Types

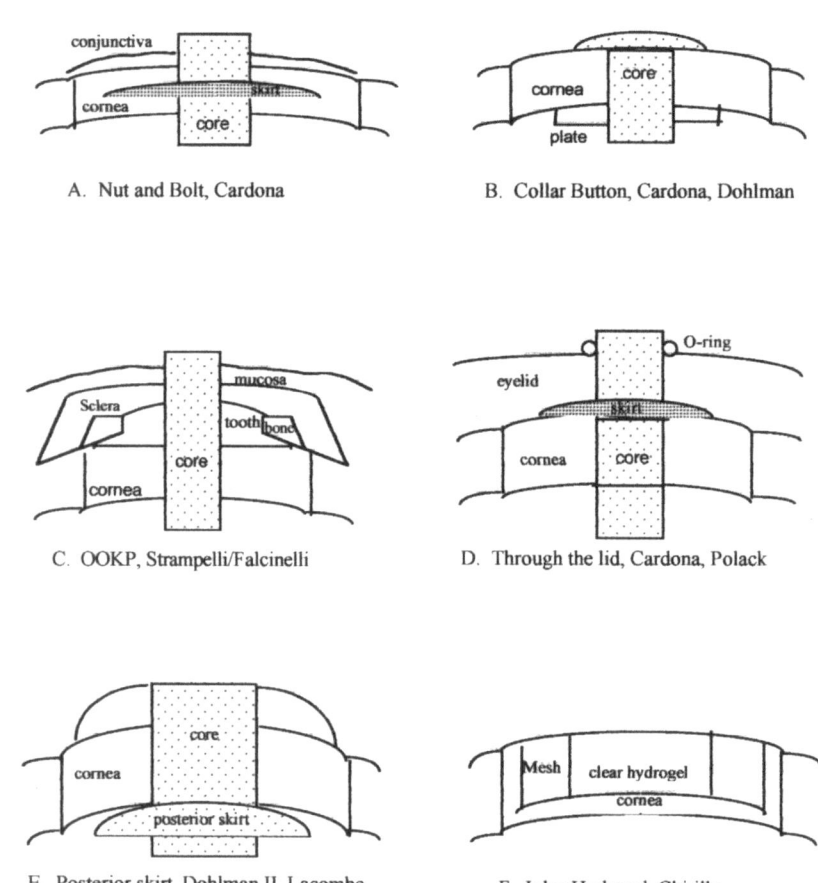

Figure 1 Schematic drawings of keratoprosthesis design types. A=Nut and bolt type, B= Collar button type, C= Osteo-odonto-keratoprosthesis, D= Through-the-lid type, E= Posterior skirt type, F= Inlay hydrogel type.

In 1962, Roper-Hall[11] implanted 6 small keratoprostheses of this design manufactured of PMMA, (Figure 1, A) but all extruded within a few months. He then started to use the Choyce modified "monoblock" (Perspex CQ) prosthesis which was one piece and had a larger core and skirt. Of forty-nine implants, one has been retained for over thirty-three years with good vision while sixteen spontaneously extruded within months. Seven of the forty-nine patients developed glaucoma, three had retinal detachments and three developed endophthalmitis. Surgical repairs were needed in thirty-three cases. Only five of these forty-nine implanted prostheses were retained more than ten years. This ten percent incidence of retention is lower than with later prostheses.

Girard[12] developed a prosthesis of the nut and bolt type (Figure 1,A) that had a fixed optical core attached to a Dacron® mesh skirt. He placed the mesh on the anterior surface of the cornea and covered it with a donor sclera which was sewn to the cornea. The PMMA core extended through the cornea posteriorly into the anterior chamber and anteriorly through the sclera overlay. He then covered the sclera and the tip of the prosthesis core with conjunctiva.

After healing stabilized the prosthesis, the conjunctiva over the core was removed to allow vision. The Dacron® mesh was intended to remain permanently, but eventually extruded through the avascular scleral graft after varying periods of time[13].

Cardona[14], working with Devoe and Castroviejo, developed a mushroom-shaped or "collar-button" type of prosthesis (Figure 1,B). The stem of the mushroom was introduced through a full-thickness hole in the cornea. A posterior plate was threaded onto the stem from the posterior side of the cornea and tightened. This prosthesis enjoyed mixed early success but was subject to leaking, infection, formation of retroprosthesis membranes, mechanical breakdown, epithelial overgrowth, epithelial downgrowth, promotion of glaucoma and eventual extrusion[15].

Dohlman, and colleagues[16], also used a two-piece collar button prosthesis similar to the Cardona mushroom, but assembled it into an 8 mm human cornea donor button which had been preserved in glycerin (Figure 1, Type B). They attached a large posterior plate (made of plastic) to the plastic mushroom stem using acrylic cement, a snap on ridge, or both. This combination of plastic and cornea was then sewn into an 8 mm trephine opening in the cornea in the same manner as a full thickness keratoplasty. Unfortunately, the same complications occurred with this prosthesis as were reported for the Cardona prosthesis, including eventual extrusion of almost all prostheses[17]. Dohlman almost completely abandoned this design in 1973, citing the high percentage of prostheses that leaked aqueous humor due to tissue melting around the core that lead to frequent extrusion and the high rate of endophthalmitis. (Personal communication in conference with fellows in March 1973).

In the early 1960s, Strampelli [18], working in Italy, realized the need for biointegration of the prosthesis into the cornea and developed the osteo-odonto-keratoprosthesis. He made use of the knowledge that the osteo-odonto ligament holds in place a relatively inert structure, a tooth, which protrudes from the surrounding tissue. Unless damaged by infection, this ligament between tooth and bone is relatively impervious to enzymatic or other degradation. To form the osteo-odonto-keratoprosthesis, Strampelli had a dentist remove one of the patient's canine teeth within a surrounding portion the jaw bone. He cut a cross-section through this specimen perpendicular to the axis of the tooth. This included bone, osteo-odonto ligament and the tooth. The cross-section was used to form a bridge between tissue and an optical core glued into the tooth (Figure 1, C). Tissue would grow into the cancellus bone. The periodontal ligament holds the tooth in the bone, stabilizing the prosthesis in the eye. When a short core was used, the eyelid would close over the prosthesis, while a long core could be extended through the eyelid, which had usually been made adherent to the eyeball. Although the periodontal ligament held the tooth firmly to the bone, there was concern about future absorption of the bone over time. This was the prosthesis that Falcinelli later revised[19].

The osteo-odonto-keratoprosthesis just described was particularly effective in cases of ocular cicatricial pemphigoid in which the disease causes the eyelid to attach to the eyeball by adhesions. Through-the-lid prostheses can cause problems, however. In 1980 Polack and Heimke[20], and in 1987 Kozarsky and colleagues[21] reported on a number of keratoprosthesis implantations they had performed using a porous ceramic skirt to promote biointegration. This prosthesis proved to be too rigid and tended to be extruded by tissue necrosis (or melting), and infection, especially when it was implanted through the eyelid (Figure 1, D).

Pintucci and colleagues[22] also used an extended prosthesis core that protruded through the eyelid and found that infection was a significant complication of this type of prosthesis. They recommended against use of a through-the-lid prosthesis.

In 1980, this author reported that a new vitreous carbon/Teflon® alloplastic material, Proplast®, was well accepted by the rabbit cornea[23]. There was fibroblastic and neovascular growth into the material but no giant cell foreign body reaction. This led to use of Proplast® as a skirt material for a core and skirt prosthesis with the skirt being inserted into an intralamellar corneal pocket and the core passing through a full thickness hole in the central cornea[24], (Figure 1, A).

After Proplast® was shown to incorporate into corneal stroma, Girard added a thin layer of Proplast® over the Dacron® net of the prosthesis that he was using. Girard found the addition of Proplast® to enhance retention of the prosthesis.[13]

Legeais, and Parisian coworkers[25], after trying three different materials, in 1993, reported initial favorable results of implanting a keratoprosthesis with a skirt made of expanded polytetrafluoroethylene (ePTFE, Gore-Tex®) (Figure 1, A)[26]. This material promoted fibrovascular invasion, which stabilization of the prosthesis. After several years, however, the fibrovascular tissue decolonized from the ePTFE, which led to loosening of the prosthesis and eventual extrusion[27].

Realizing the need for a readily available synthetic material which would integrate biologically, Pintucci and Pintucci[28], studied the work of DeBakey on vascular replacement using Dacron® materials. They then designed a keratoprosthesis with a Dacron® felt skirt (Figure 1, A) that they implanted under the lower eyelid for two months so that it would biocolonize with the patient's own tissues. After removing the buried implant, excess tissue was trimmed from the skirt and it was sewn to the anterior surface of the cornea. It was covered with mucosa from either the back of the lower lip or the hard palate. The hard palate mucosa proved more effective in extremely dry eyes[29].

Worst[30], focusing on designing a keratoprosthesis that would create improved mechanical stability, developed a prosthesis shaped like a round head rivet (Figure 1, B). The domed anterior end had four holes around the edge through which stainless steel sutures were placed to anchor the prosthesis to the rectus muscles or the sclera in front of them. The shaft of the rivet was introduced through a hole made through and through the cornea. There was no posterior plate or flange. The design relied on the stainless steel sutures to hold the prosthesis tightly in place, to prevent leakage from the eye, and to transmit the mechanical forces impinging on the prosthesis onto the eye. Worst later modified his prosthesis, making the core conical. The larger diameter end of the cone formed the posterior surface of the prosthesis and the smaller diameter end attached to the center of the optical cap[31]. He called this his "Champagne cork" prosthesis.

Singh[32] reported on use of a keratoprosthesis of modified Worst design. Singh's design, which resembles an automobile wheel rim with a hubcap on the anterior surface, was also held in place with wire sutures from the anterior rim[32].

Dohlman, because of frequent failures with the original two piece prosthesis, (C.H. Dohlman, MD Keratoprosthesis: Dohlman-Doane Types I and II Research Instructions, Boston, 1994) designed a two piece "sandwich" type of prosthesis having a mushroom-shaped core, 3 mm in diameter, with an anterior cap, 7 mm in diameter, that overlaps the cornea by two millimeters peripheral to the core. It has a posterior plate, a 9 mm round titanium disk, fenestrated with 16 small holes[33], (Figure 1, E). This prosthesis is assembled into a donor cornea, similar to his original prosthesis. The donor cornea is then sewn into the recipient as a routine corneal transplant would be. This prosthesis relies on mechanical forces to hold it in place.

Several other polymers have been studied for their biointegration properties. Kim, and coworkers.[34] studied four fibrous polymers (polypropylene, two kinds of polyethylene terephthalate, and polyurethane). They concluded that polypropylene had better biological stability for a keratoprosthesis. The result of their efforts is the Seoul-type prosthesis with a fibrous polypropylene skirt (Figure 1, A). This prosthesis is currently under evaluation.

In 1997, Chirila[35], working in Perth, Australia, reported a novel prosthesis design that used a poly hydroxyethyl methacrylate (PHEMA) hydrogel material used for both the smooth, clear, optical central disk and a porous mesh ring that would allow for biointegration of the periphery of the prosthesis. The fused two-part prosthesis is a large disk approximately as thick as the corneal. It is sutured into the cornea in the same manner as corneal tissue in a routine deep anterior lamellar keratoplasty, (Figure 1, F). It is being studied for biointegration of the porous portion and maintenance of an epithelial covering over the central clear portion.

Caldwell[36] has developed a similar prosthesis using a type of urethane for the optical portions and a fibrous haptic ring with radial strips that are imbedded in the sclera. The two parts are bonded with proprietary glue. He has studied this prosthesis in monkeys and a few human patients.

There is growing acceptance, among investigators, of the need for biointegration between the prosthesis and the surrounding tissue. Several synthetic fibrous materials that promote biointegration are now under trials. I feel that, to be successful, the prosthesis must have both biointegration and mechanical stability, including a proper distribution of the forces directed at the prosthesis.

To facilitate the incorporation of porous materials into the cornea to anchor a prosthesis, Trinkaus-Randell[37] studied keratocyte seeding of porous polypropylene disks, *in vivo*, to enhance fibroplasia and collagen deposition within the pores.

Over the years, the search for a material to hold the prosthesis core in the cornea have included, celluloid, egg membranes, tooth and bone, bone, acrylic, Plexiglas, Teflon®, ceramic, hydroxyappetite, Proplast®, ePTFE, Dacron® felt, PHEMA hydrogel, and fibrous polypropylene. Only tooth and bone, ePTFE, Dacron® felt, PHEMA hydrogel, polypropylene, and aliphatic polyether based urethane are now being used.

Part Four

Causes for Prosthesis Failure

The literature is replete with reports of early success with keratoprostheses of novel design. However, the late complications and failures of these prostheses often do not get reported in the literature. Long term studies of success or failure are rare. When the failures are reported, usually as unpublished papers given at meetings, the problems which lead to these failures are consistent, from one prosthesis to another[15]. The causes of prosthesis failure consistently fall into two major categories: the mechanical forces working the prosthesis loose or biomedical factors causing tissue melting, infection, glaucoma or retroprosthetic membranes.

Mechanical Causes of Keratoprosthesis Failure Mechanical causes for failure of a prosthesis are those that derive from the design of the prosthesis to tissue interface, mechanical failure of the prosthesis itself (breakage), failure to respect the forces which apply to the prosthesis (intraocular pressure, lid movement, and globe movement), and mechanical results of biomedical failures (loss of support).

Globe movement problems are greatest when the prosthesis is placed through the eyelid without immobilizing the eyelid by creating adhesions between the eyelid and the eyeball. Adhesions would bind the eye and eyelid together, decreasing the movements that create great stress on the tissue surrounding the core and any parts that are attached to the core and to the eyeball.

Eyelid movement over or against a short core or pulling on a long, through-the-lid core creates repeated trauma to the prosthesis and the cornea, working the prosthesis loose, promoting leakage or extrusion.

One of the forces that impinge on a prosthesis is intraocular pressure. Although intraocular pressure is essential for maintenance of the shape of the eye, this same force exerts constant pressure on the prosthesis to push it from the cornea. Intraocular pressure puts force on the posterior surfaces of the prosthesis. This force is transmitted by the prosthesis onto the corneal tissue. Uneven distribution of the force, or a prosthesis design that localizes the pressure in small areas (skirt too small, too rigid, too floppy, or with a small edge area), may lead to pressure necrosis.

Applying hydraulic principles, we know that the total force that intraocular pressure places on the prosthesis is proportional to the surface area of the opening into the eye through which the core passes. The force is directed along a vector centripetal to the ocular center. For equilibrium and stability to be maintained, this pressure must be counteracted by an equal and opposite force from the cornea onto the prosthesis. ($F = MA$, If A, [movement] $= 0$, then ΣF must $= 0$)

The earlier prostheses had small intralamellar disks or skirts that were thought to be the cause of pressure necrosis of the cornea. The total force exerted on an exposed area equals the force per unit of area times the total area exposed. The area is calculated from the radius by the formula πr^2 while the perimeter (circumference), which is the area of contact for a floppy skirt, is calculated by the formula $2\pi r$. For a rigid, well fitting skirt the formula for the area of diffusion of the forces is $\pi r_1^2 - \pi r_2^2$ where r_1 is the outer radius of the skirt and r_2 is the radius of the hole in the cornea for the core. While the circumference increases linearly with the radius, the area increases exponentially. If the width of the skirt, transmitting the force, remains constant at 2 millimeters, the total area of the skirt will increase with increasing core radius, better diffusing the increasing force from intraocular pressure applied to the core over a larger skirt area. Increasing the skirt width further decreases the force per unit area that must be transmitted to the cornea. Very large skirts, however, will thicken the peripheral cornea and interfere with the angle structures, causing glaucoma, which, in turn, increases the force to expel the implant. With the appropriate rigidity of the skirt material and good biointegration, the force is transmitted to the entire area of the cornea in contact with the skirt (πr^2 for the skirt minus πr^2 for the core opening). Because of the forward vector of the force, a flexible skirt will not transmit the force beyond the core edge. Conversely, a very rigid skirt may transmit the force to one particular spot or a ring on the cornea.

Table1. Ratios of Forces on the Prosthesis to Supporting Areas of the Cornea, Based on Radius of the Core

Radius of core (r)	1mm	2mm	3mm	4mm	5mm	6mm
Area of Core (A) or (Pr)	3.14	12.56	28.26	50.24	78.50	113.04
Circumference of core (C)	6.28	12.56	18.84	25.12	31.40	37.68
Ratio of A:C	0.50	1.00	1.50	2.00	2.50	3.00
Area of 2mm skirt (S)	12.56	37.68	50.24	62.80	75.36	87.92
Ratio of Areas S:P	4:1	3:1	1.77:1	1.25:1	0.96:1	0.78:1

Table 1. r = radius of the core; A or Pr = Area or Relative pressure from the posterior surface of the core; C = Circumference of the core; Ratio A:C = Relation of the cross section area to the linear circumference of the core; 2 mm Rim area, S = Area of a 2 mm wide skirt with relation to the radius of the core; Ratio Areas S:P = Comparison of attachment zone area of the cornea(S) to the exposed surface area of core bearing the intraocular pressure(P).

A comparison of the area of the skirt to the area of the core (the ratio S/P in Table 1) shows that a core with a diameter of 2 mm has a ratio of 4:1 ratio, or the area of the skirt with good force dispersion to the area of the core. This ratio becomes 1.25:1 for a core with a diameter of 4 mm (Table 1). The 5 and 6 mm cores have more than 1 mm^2 of support area for each unit of pressure. To obtain an even more favorable ratio, it is necessary to increase the width of the skirt, impinging on the peripheral cornea and angle structures.

A comparison of these ratios demonstrates that the larger the core is, the more force is exerted on the skirt. Smaller cores do have the advantage of leaving more room in the cornea for biointegration of wider skirts to decrease the force per unit area on the skirt. Cores of 4 to 5 mm diameter allow large skirts and thus transmit less force per unit area of contact between the skirt and the cornea. On the other hand, cores larger than 5 mm in diameter create larger forces on the core to distribute through a smaller remaining skirt area.

Materials with uneven thickness that are imbedded in the cornea may cause localized anterior displacement of the overlying cornea (bumps). These bumps will in turn cause pressure necrosis with erosion of the tissue over the area of the bump[22].

To diffuse the pressure evenly without causing local pressure points, the skirt material must be of sufficient rigidity to spread the force over the entire area. Flexible skirt material will cause all of the pressure to be borne by the tissue at the junction between the rigid core and the flexible skirt. If the skirt is rigid, but does not conform perfectly to the same shape as the corneal tissue, pressure will be transmitted to a point or points of local contact. The ideal skirt material must have the proper rigidity to transmit the forces while being flexible enough to avoid localized pressure points.

Biointegration of the prosthesis into the supporting tissue helps to diffuse the forces from the prosthesis to the supporting tissue. The Chirila[36] prosthesis promotes peripheral integration for almost the full thickness of the corneal with a large area of contact because it has a large diameter. Posterior pressure on this prosthesis is also decreased by leaving Descemet's membrane and some posterior stroma intact behind the prosthesis to contain some of the force produced by intraocular pressure.

Worst[30,] van Andel[31,] and Singh[32] use stainless-steel sutures to anchor the prosthesis to the sclera or extra-ocular muscles by mechanical force. One common cause of failure of this Prosthesis is metal fatigue of the stainless steel sutures. Another cause of failure is the dissection of the steel sutures through tissues, because of the forces they transmit. Singh found that if she used steel sutures to encircle the globe to anchor the prosthesis, the wire eventually cut through the sclera into the ocular contents. She reports a case of in which the retina is draped over the stainless steel suture that has cut through the back of the eye.

The new Dohlman prosthesis[33], because of its large size, can transmit a large force to the surrounding corneal tissue. The small diameter of the core in this prosthesis and the large area of contact between the prosthesis and the cornea, afforded by the titanium plate that extends behind the peripheral cornea, allow a large area for diffusion of pressure. This prosthesis, due to its size and shape, does encroach upon the angle, which is probably what causes most cases of glaucoma associated with the use of this prosthesis. Glaucoma increases the total force with which the flange pushes against the cornea. This force is decreased by the mandatory placement of a glaucoma drain and reservoir at the time of prosthesis insertion.

Many prostheses of early design had a significant failure rate from breakage of the prosthesis. Back plates became unscrewed, glues failed, snap on plates became unsnapped, and plates cracked and became loose. Cores separated from skirts and other forms of attachment.

Early prostheses were made by hand and then hand polished. It is commendable that the optics worked as well as they did. The state of the art with the contact lens swing lathe and polishing equipment enable the production of prostheses with contact lens quality optics.

In fact, the desire to create a prosthesis with accurate optical power was one reason for Cardona[2] to design the nut and bolt prosthesis with a system to adjust the optical power by adjusting the height of the core, thereby changing the optical length of the eye. He placed two small holes in the front surface of the core. A spanner wrench like tool was introduced into these holes to screw the core in or out to adjust the optical length of the eye to focus the image on the retina. Unfortunately, when core height was adjusted to correct for optical errors, the core became too recessed, allowing conjunctival overgrowth, or too elevated, causing repeated bumping of the core by the eyelid. However, the visual improvement from most prostheses is so great for the patients that they do not mind wearing spectacles to correct small errors in refraction that were uncorrected by the prosthesis.

Dohlman uses a soft bandage lens over the prosthesis to protect the eye and keep the front of the eye wet[33]. Corrective power can be added by this contact lens, if needed.

Biological Causes of Prosthesis Failure Biological causes of prosthesis failure have become better understood as more has been learned about corneal biochemistry, the activity and inhibition of enzymes, corneal vascularization, activities of the proteins in serum, and the growing host of biological and alloplastic materials used in implants.

Most early researchers in the field of keratoprostheses did not consider biological causes of failure and instead attributed all failures to mechanical design. Prostheses were extruded because of "pressure necrosis" or infection.

Retroprosthesis membranes formed and contracted, causing the prosthesis to extrude. Fortunately, when this happened, the membrane usually prevented loss of contents from the globe and some vision remained.

When the prostheses leaked because of "melting" at the tissue prosthesis interface, the eye became hypotonic and then eventually developed choroidal edema or retinal detachment or it became infected. The infection usually progressed to endophthalmitis with resultant loss of the eye or at least all potential for vision.

When I studied failed and failing prostheses made of PMMA, it became apparent that the interface between cornea and the parts made of PMMA was not stable. Initially the loss of tissue around the prosthesis was thought to be simple necrosis[38]. Because of the work of Turss and colleagues[39], and D. M. Maurice, MD, Ph.D. (2000 Castroviejo Society Lecture, Orlando, Florida), it was found that dissolution of tissue around the core is probably due to poor corneal nutrition. Thoft and co-workers[40] showed that the cornea receives water, glycogen, and proteins from the aqueous humor and becomes necrotic when these are blocked. A posterior plastic plate or membrane has been shown to block this flow of water and nutrition into the cornea.

In about 1970, Slansky and colleagues[41] and Berman and colleagues[42] reported that corneal melting was caused by collagenase and also determined that the open edge of corneal epithelium was the source of this collagenase. The collagenase can diffuse under the front plate of a prosthesis, digesting the stromal collagen.

With many early Dohlman prostheses, dissolution of the corneal tissue around the core led to slow leaks that could be demonstrated by Seidel testing. Placing chips of donor cornea around the core could close these leaks temporarily, but the chips soon dissolved. It was also noted that those corneas which were heavily vascularized to the edge of the optical core did not melt and remained stable. This was consistent with the clinical observations that atrophic corneas which melted to become deep ulcers stopped melting in areas where the cornea became vascularized. Once the cornea is totally vascularized, it is nourished and the enzymes that would dissolve it are inhibited by the serum proteins which diffused into the stroma[43].

The weak point for failure, where the tissue meets the alloplastic material, requires a material–biological or alloplastic–that will allow fusion of the optical system of the prosthesis and the tissue of the host, or at least that it will prevent dissolution of the cornea.

Dohlman and colleagues[44] demonstrated that corneal melting at the edges of chronic epithelial defects could be prevented by removing all epithelium and then gluing PMMA disks similar to contact lenses to the corneal stroma using n-haptyl methyl methacrylate adhesive (Histocryl Blau, Firma Braun, Melsingen, Germany). The PMMA disk and glue blocked enzymes from the stroma. Unfortunately, all of these barrier lenses became loose or detached, allowing further melting.

Slansky and colleagues[41] showed that either a 1 molar solution of ethylenediaminetetraacetic acid (EDTA) or either a 10 or 20% solution of methyl cystiene (Mucomyst) would inhibit corneal collagenase. Medroxyprogesterone (Provera®) eye drops also retard collagenase activity[45].

At about the same time that Slansky and Berman and colleagues were studying collagenase activity, the pulmonary disease resulting from alpha-1-antitrypsin deficiency was becoming well defined. Lieberman[46] described a deficiency of alpha-1-antitrypsin, a major inhibitor/regulator of collagenase activity that allowed major collagenase damage to occur to the lungs. He stated that alpha-2-macroglobulin has an even stronger, non reversible, inhibiting effect on collagenase.

An investigation was done, using time-exposure fluorescent photography techniques and fluorescein labeled antibodies to study the distribution of both alpha-1-antitrypsin (α-1-at) and alpha-2-macroglobulin (α-2-mg) in human corneas. It demonstrated that α-1-at was distributed throughout the stroma, epithelium, and endothelium, but was relatively absent in Bowman's and Descemet's layers. Alpha-2-mg was not found in normal cornea, probably due to the large size of the molecule. In sections from chronically vascularized corneas, α-2-mg was found in the cornea within 500 microns of blood vessels (unpublished data, 1973). This is consistent with the work of Stock and Aronson[47] on immune globulin distribution in the cornea. The presence of α-2-mg near vessels would explain how vascularization of the cornea or a prosthesis skirt provides inhibition of collagenase.

Berman[48] and others, who have studied metalo-collagenases, have found that their activation depends on the plasmin activation cascade. This discovery has opened the way to develop new means of inhibition of collagenase, based on interruption of the plasmin cascade. Although important in the understanding of prosthesis retention, this field is too vast to consider in greater depth here.

No prosthesis reported on to date can support total corneal epithelial coverage of a permanent nature. Intact epithelium is a major barrier to all but a few bacteria, while absence of this barrier invites bacterial invasion. Wherever epithelium borders on hard plastic there is lack of epithelial continuity and opportunity for bacterial invasion. In patients receiving steroids and eyes without adequate vascularization, the corneal milieu promotes growth by some bacteria or fungi and allows collagenase activity. Collagenase is also produced by some bacteria, particularly *Pseudomonas* species, and by neutrophils. The latter release the collagenase they produce at sites of inflammation.

Once there is sufficient enzymatic degradation of the collagen, leakage of aqueous humor develops, creating hypotony and allowing migration of the bacteria into the eye. The final result is usually retinal detachment or endophthalmitis. This chain of events is particularly common with through-the-eyelid prostheses. The eyelid obstructs the view of the developing problems in the deeper layers and within the globe, delaying diagnosis, thereby adding to the severity of the infection. Constant mechanical trauma from attempted eyelid or eyeball movement creates pathways for bacterial invasion.

Even when there is no mechanical problem with the prosthesis or biological problem, such as collagen melting, conjunctival or mucosal retraction, or infection, vision may be obstructed and anterior displacement of the prosthesis may occur because of formation of a membrane across the back of the optical core. This retroprosthetic membrane is fibrous in nature and may vascularize. Over time, the membrane contracts, shortening the distance from the corneal edges around the posterior extension of the optical core. Normal biological shrinkage of the membrane pushes the optical core forward and the pulls posterior corneal lamella posteriorly, away from the skirt material, thereby loosening the prosthesis. Bath[49] reported that opening or removing the membrane surgically, or by laser, is sometimes followed by recurrence of the membrane.

Another frequent cause of prosthesis failure is epithelial downgrowth along the prosthesis core or around the skirt into the anterior chamber[50]. The subsequent spread of epithelium throughout the anterior chamber blocks aqueous outflow, causing intractable glaucoma. The epithelial tract is also a path of leakage of the aqueous humor from the eye and a route for bacterial invasion of the eye. If the epithelium lines the hole through the cornea, the hole will not close and heal. Thus, blockage of epithelial growth into the prosthesis and the surrounding tissue is an important goal of prosthesis design and implantation technique.

Placement of some of the prosthetic designs has required removal of the crystalline lens and the iris along with the anterior vitreous. The inflammation caused by removing these structures poses high risk for glaucoma and the growth of retroprosthetic membranes. Glaucoma is so prevalent that some surgeons routinely place a glaucoma drain and reservoir in the eye when implanting a prosthesis[51]. In patients with glaucoma due to a prosthesis, the prosthesis prevents effective use of most instruments for measuring intraocular pressure. Small optical cores also restrict visual fields, which removes one of the methods of evaluation of glaucoma progression.[52]

Part Five

Design Solutions for Prosthesis Problems

Many variations on early prosthesis designs have been proposed to solve one or more problems with these devices. Some modifications have shown promise in improving prosthesis retention or design, but others can be discarded. Examination of success factors related to each part of the prosthesis and of the many variations proposed for that part should lead to an optimal design for a keratoprosthesis.

Prosthesis Core The core is the heart of any prosthesis. It must be sturdy, optically correct, stable, and provide a useful visual field while causing a minimum of problems.

Early optical cores were cylindrical, 2 to 3 mm in diameter and 6 to 8 mm long[2,10,38]. These dimensions limited the visual field, theoretically, to about 30 degrees and required removal of the crystalline lens from the eye to make room for the posterior extension of the core extending through the anterior chamber.

Hille and colleagues[52], from Germany, presented the results of implanting osteo-odonto-keratoprostheses with cores of various lengths and diameters into several patients. They found that the measured visual field was actually smaller than the theoretical field size in patients who had implants with cores 3.0 and 3.5 mm diameter and 7 to 8 mm long. Actual fields were 20 degrees for eyes with 3.0 mm cores and 50 degrees for eyes with implants with 3.5 mm cores. This compared to predicted fields of 55 and 65 degrees respectively. Using ray-tracing they found a theoretical field of 140 degrees with implants of 4.5 mm diameter that were 4 mm long. By calculating the fields for various lengths and diameters of implants, they found that field increased faster with decreases in core length than it did with increases in core diameter. They postulated that the difference between theoretical and actual fields was caused by internal reflection from the core walls and imperfect centering and alignment of the core axis with the retina. Cardona[53] etched the walls of the core to reduce internal reflections, but did not say anything about visual field size of his patients.

Through-the-eyelid prostheses require longer cores to pass through the thickness of the eyelid. The osteo-odonto-keratoprosthesis must use a long core because of the thickness of the bone and tooth skirt. Use of a thin synthetic skirt material allows the core to be shorter, thus resulting in a larger visual field. An optical core diameter of 4.5 or 5.0 mm with a length of 6 mm or less in length should give a useful visual field.

Hull and co-workers[54], in London, found that their patients with prostheses also had decreased fields, which they thought were caused by decreased retinal luminance through the optical core and other optical aberrations. They suggested four ways to increase visual field:

1. Increase the posterior diameter of the core
2. Accept a certain degree of myopia
3. Use a multiple-lens system, or
4. Shortening the length of the core

Recent studies with intraocular lenses have demonstrated that decreased visual acuity may be due to the reduction of contrast sensitivity caused by the lens plastic[55]. This could also explain the decreased visual field and visual acuity through prostheses.

In 1991, at the Keratoprosthesis study Group meeting in Rome, both Worst[30] and Barber[56] reported new prosthesis core designs. Both designs used increasing core diameter from anterior to posterior to produce a theoretically enlarged visual field and increased core stability. The Worst "champagne cork" prosthesis had a curved front optical surface cap attached in one piece to a conical core that increased from a 3 mm in diameter at the base of the cap to a 5 mm diameter at the posterior flat end.

The Barber design, called the "lighthouse", had a 6.0 mm diameter anterior curved optical surface, with a 60 diopter spherical end surface, that was continued posteriorly as a 5 mm diameter cylindrical core that extended 1.5 mm before becoming conical for 4 mm to end in a 6 mm diameter round, flat, posterior surface. The entire prosthesis was 6.0 mm in length, including the anterior curved optical surface.

Prosthesis cores that are conical should theoretically provide a larger visual field. The conical shape has a second advantage because the increasing diameter of the core forces the 4.5 mm hole in the posterior corneal lamella forward, up the cone and against the skirt.

The presently preferred core material in hard core prostheses is intraocular lens quality PMMA[57] This material is biochemically stabile and has shown good compatibility with eye tissues.

The author has implanted a prosthesis with a soft silicone optical core in cat eyes. The core became hazy after several months and haze matured with time. (Unpublished data) Newer intraocular lenses of foldable acrylate or silicone do not have this problem, but these materials have not been tried in a keratoprosthesis for clinical use.

Worst continues to implant prostheses made with glass or polycarbonate cores that are manufactured by Philips' Optics[30]. According to Worst, glass is preferable to plastic for the core because it is more resistant to scratching.

Chirila's prosthesis has a core of hydrogel material[35] that is pliable and remains clear for long periods. It is somewhat impermeable to water and nutrients so it does not support an epithelial surface well. It is placed in a deep stromal bed, avoiding the problem of retroprosthesis membrane development. The prosthesis is implanted by sewing it into the cornea using the same procedure as a lamellar corneal transplant.

The most recent prosthesis, reported by Caldwell[36], in 1997, is called "The Soft Keratoprosthesis." He has conducted a series of implantations in animals to develop a thin curved device which is flush with the sclera. This prosthesis uses a soft elastomeric optic (aliphatic polyether-based urethane) which is bonded by heated pressurized injection molding to a 60 mμ porous polytetrafluoroethylene skirt. He describes six radial strip haptics which are embedded in the sclera for biocolonization. Caldwell claims better acceptance with fewer complications along with better cosmetic appearance and better visual field.

Caldwell has reported studies in two human subjects with prostheses which developed complications, especially when a detailed post operative medication routine was allowed to lapse. His major problems were retroprosthetic membranes, epithelial downgrowth, separation at the optic/skirt junction, collagen melting, and endophthalmitis. He tried a new prosthesis with supposed better optic/skirt binding in three monkeys with good results, but he has not reported further studies with this prosthesis.

The new Dohlman collar-button prosthesis[33] is constructed of polymerized PMMA and a posterior titanium plate. It has curved anterior and posterior plates with surface curves similar to the natural cornea. The posterior plate extends behind the cornea and is very near the iris plane and angle structures. There is no biointegration of this prosthesis.

The optical power required in any prosthesis core differs depending on whether the crystalline lens is removed or left in place. Short Cores in phakic eyes (lens still in the eye) usually are made with 45 diopters of power while aphakic eyes usually require 60 diopters of power to compensate for the lens removal. Most prosthesis designers have found it convenient to place the optical power on the anterior surface and to make the posterior surface flat. Variations on the curvatures of the front and back surfaces or the use of two elements in the core lens could theoretically give better visual fields and image sizes, but little work has been done on these refinements.

If the core protrudes to far above the outer surface, movement of the eyelid causes repeated trauma to the eyelid and the prosthesis, that leads to tissue necrosis or mechanical loosening. If the core does not protrude far enough above the surface, the conjunctival covering the cornea tends to grow over the core and block the optical path. This can be managed by trimming tissue back from the core from time to time[15], but is a nuisance and increases the chance of infection.

Long posterior protrusion requires removal of the lens and iris. The resultant collapse of the angle structures and the inflammation caused by this surgery may be the cause of glaucoma seen in these prosthesis patients. Longer protrusion was thought to decrease the formation of retroprosthesis membranes, but this has not been proven. Retroprosthetic membranes, unless removed promptly, can cause extrusion of the prosthesis.

It was originally thought that the membranes would not form if the core extended far enough into the anterior chamber. However, it may be that core shape plays a more important role than core length in membrane formation. The conical core, expanding posteriorly, creates an acute angle between the core and skirt, which should cause edge inhibition of the endothelium and hold the posterior corneal lamella forward, against the skirt. Shape may not be the only important cause, because inflammation caused by surgery or infection, with the production of plasmoid aqueous and fibrin, may play a more significant role in membrane formation.

Worst[30] had no retroprosthetic membranes in 42 PMMA prostheses, 5 membranes in 29 glass prostheses (17%) and 2 membranes in 35 polycarbonate prostheses (6%). Cardona and Dohlman have both found a high incidence of retroprosthetic membranes with straight PMMA cores.

Prosthesis flanges and skirts To prevent conjunctiva from extending over the optical core, Cardona placed O-rings in a grove at the anterior end of the core. O-rings were effective but proved impractical because of the eyelid action striking the core and pushing the ring loose, usually with loss of the tiny ring.

This author reported use of an anterior flange that was created by making the anterior surface diameter of the prosthesis 1 mm larger than the core diameter, producing a 0.5 mm overhang or flange[55]. A trial of this implant in cats demonstrated that a fixed flange that is slightly above the surface of the conjunctiva that had been advanced to cover the corneal surface, prevents the conjunctiva from growing up and over the core. The thin edge and the extended curvature of the anterior surface serves to guide the eyelid over the prosthesis with less mechanical stress than when the eyelid hits the protruding perpendicular edge of the core without a flange. An elevation of 0.5 mm above the corneal surface was shown in this prior trial to give adequate room for the conjunctiva to cover the cornea under the flange without core protrusion to the height of interference with the eyelid.

Placement of the optical core itself into the cornea, with or without attempts at support, was tried in the very early designs, but the dissolution of the tissue around the core allowed the core to become loose and extrude. A simple core placed in the cornea also allowed the epithelium to grow along the opening into the anterior chamber. This led to infection or intractable glaucoma with loss of the eye. A lateral extension of the implant onto, into or behind the cornea as a flange or skirt was thought necessary to hold the optical portion and to prevent early extrusion.

Anterior and posterior plates on the surfaces of the cornea, as used in the Cardona and early Dohlman prostheses, might theoretically also block enzymes from reaching the corneal stroma while holding the core in place. In the clinical situation, with the unavoidable movement of the prosthesis and plasticity of the tissue, the enzymes do reach the prosthesis/tissue interface, allowing enzymatic degradation of the tissue and loss of support for the prosthesis. This has been reported with most simple prostheses.

Large solid plastic skirts within or behind the cornea did not work well. Cornea tissue that was anterior to a wide solid skirt did not maintain epithelium and was susceptible to enzymatic degradation. Turss, Friend and Dohlman[38] demonstrated that impermeable membranes placed between deep corneal lamellae or behind the cornea caused central epithelial defects and central corneal necrosis. We now know that nutrition moves through the cornea from the anterior chamber, perpendicular to the corneal surface, with very little lateral diffusion. D. M. Maurice, MD (2000 Castroviejo Society Lecture, Orlando, Florida) reported that the extent of lateral diffusion in the cornea is less than 1 mm when the blocking material is at the posterior depth of the cornea.

Solid skirts more than 1 mm wider than the core, without pores or openings cause necrosis of the unnourished cornea with corneal melting beyond the lateral diffusion area anterior to the plate. Cornea anterior to a solid flange or skirt will also not maintain an epithelium causing release of collagenase from the epithelial edge and allowing infection through the epithelial defect. In the early Dohlman prosthesis, if the grafted cornea between the plates became vascularized to the edge of the core, the tissue did not dissolve and the epithelium would cover any exposed cornea. Corneal nutrition was provided by the vascular bed.

Prosthesis designers began making fenestrations in solid intralamellar skirts of the prostheses with the stated intent of allowing healing (scarring) to develop through the holes. Girard[24] used an open net skirt of different materials, usually Dacron®, to promote scarring with fibrous entanglement of the skirt. These designs allowed better nutrition for the anterior layers, but did not lead to better tissue integration. Solid skirts have been replaced in most prostheses by porous fibrous materials or fenestrated solid plates.

The recurring problems of melting and extrusion, with the related complications of leakage, and epithelial downgrowth with subsequent glaucoma and infection, led to a realization of the need for integration between the prosthesis and the surrounding tissues. Integration between tissue and prosthesis creates a barrier to epithelium and bacteria and provides more stability for the prosthesis.

Strampelli[18] used a slice of bone and tooth, cut perpendicular to the axis of the tooth such that the cross section of tooth was held in the bone by the periodontal ligament. A hole was drilled through the tooth, into which the plastic optical core was cemented. The combination of bone and tooth created a biological skirt which could heal to the cornea by fibrovascular invasion of the porous bone. This prosthesis, with modifications by Falcinelli[19], has proven to be one of the most stable prostheses to date, but it still has limitations.

The need for better biointegration of keratoprosthesis has prompted the search for a more readily available alloplastic material that will allow biointegration and stability similar to the bone and tooth skirt.

The acceptance and biointegration of Proplast® into rabbit cornea has been reported[23]. Proplast® was found to stimulate vascularization from the limbus with invasion of fibrovascular tissue into the interstices of the material. It did not incite a foreign body, giant cell granuloma response. Once the Proplast® had become incorporated into the cornea it was not possible to remove it without destroying the Proplast and the cornea. The pore size of Proplast® is large enough to permit in-growth of fibroblasts and vessels. The carbon fibers of Proplast® are wettable, which allows the cells to attach to produce a stable interface.

When thin disks of Proplast®, (0.25 or 0.3 mm thickness), were placed in lamellar pockets in the rabbit cornea, the Proplast® vascularized from the limbus in 3 to 4 weeks and there were large areas of biointegration. Disks with thick, square edges developed pressure necrosis or melting over the thick edges. Tapering of the edges prevented this necrosis and exposure of the Proplast®.

In some animals, only part of the Proplast® became invaded by fibrovascular tissue. Some sectors did not contain feeder vessels in the peripheral cornea. When animals were pretreated by placing 12 evenly spaced radial 9-0 silk sutures in the peripheral 3 mm of the cornea, the entire peripheral cornea became vascularized. Placement of Proplast® disks in lamellar pockets in these vascularized corneas led to complete fibrovascular incorporation of the implant.

Proplast® has many qualities that make it a good material for a prosthesis. It is porous and wettable so that it incorporates well. It is stiff, but not hard, so that it is forgiving concerning local pressure when properly shaped, yet it is rigid enough to transmit the forces to a wide area of contact.

Because of difficulties in obtaining the bone and tooth skirt for the osteo-odonto-keratoprosthesis from the patient's jaw, Temprano[58], in Spain, has experimented with the use of a disk of tibial bone as a biological skirt. He found that the tibial bone is absorbed over time, making this substitute unacceptable.

Ligeais and colleagues[59], in Paris, used pHEMA as a porous skirt material. They had early success with this material, but over the long term the rate of extrusion was high. They reported that, although there is the initial fibrovascular tissue invasion of the material, the new tissue later atrophies, resulting in loosening and extrusion of the keratoprosthesis.

Pintucci and colleagues[28], working in Rome, but separate from Falcinelli, have studied several types of Dacron® fabric that DeBakey had used for vascular grafts. They found that the woven fabric did not integrate well in to the cornea, but that the Dacron® felt used for aortic grafts was well incorporated in to the cornea. They also determined that thin layers (0.2 mm) encapsulate, but do not have tissue invasion, whereas layers 0.6 mm and 1.4 mm do become totally biointegrated[29]. Since the 1.4 mm layers are thinker than a cornea and they become inflexible, leading to erosion, he uses the 0.6 mm thick material. Pintucci reports on eighteen years of moderate to good success using prostheses made with Dacron® felt skirts, but he continues to have complications of infection and extrusion.

Part Six

Psychological Considerations

There are profound ethical questions involved in keratoprosthesis surgery which must be addressed by researchers and surgeons in the field. Because of the complexity of these procedures and their high failure rate, the criteria that have evolved for selection of patients to undergo surgery include significant visual impairment in both eyes. Prosthesis surgery has a high risk of total loss of vision or loss of the eye that may occur at varying intervals after implantation.

Many of the patients who undergo keratoprosthesis surgery have undergone multiple unsuccessful corneal transplants or other surgeries to restore lost vision due to a corneal disorder. These patients tend to develop a strong belief that, by the use of a corneal prosthesis that will not reject, the surgeon will bring about a permanent cure of their blindness.

Indeed, after the two or more procedures needed to implant a keratoprosthesis and the removal of tissue covering the keratoprosthesis, most patients usually do experience rapid return of significantly improved vision. Suddenly the patient, who was blind, or almost blind, can see very well again. They hold their surgeon in very high regard—a miracle worker. Then, in the hope and belief that the improvement in vision is permanent, many patients make unrealistic career choices before experiencing failure of the prosthesis and profound depression.

The ethical dilemma for the surgeon is this: We know that these prostheses are prone to failure, often earlier rather than later. Should we be offering patients a "cure" for corneal blindness that is, according to statistical probability, very likely to fail? Should we be more aggressive in counseling our patients on the tentative nature of keratoprosthesis results, or should we abandon corneal prostheses altogether until we have perfected them in animals?

Polack and colleagues[60], who implanted a keratoprosthesis with a ceramic skirt (hydroxyappetite), addressed this problem by requiring each of the patients to participate in a minimum of six hours of psychological counseling that included discussions of the possibility of failure and the life changes which could result from both success and failure of the keratoprosthesis.

They implanted fifteen through-the-lid prostheses and ten through only the cornea and conjunctiva[61]. All of the through-the-lid prostheses were lost within two years. Despite counseling and warnings, almost all of the patients became despondent after loss of the prosthesis—one patient even threatening the doctor.

I believe that patients will often self-deceive by promising the surgeon and themselves to be satisfied with any eventual outcome, if they can be allowed to have the surgery. Once the prosthesis is lost, they fail to remember their prior commitment to be satisfied that they had made the attempt, regardless of the outcome.

The other moral question involves the use of bilateral keratoprostheses in individuals who have sustained corneal blindness in both eyes. In the present status of keratoprostheses with the numerous complications often leading to the loss of all vision upon extrusion of the prosthesis or endophthalmitis, is it appropriate to put both eyes in jeopardy with keratoprostheses when the average duration of a prosthesis is less than five years? One famous prosthesis surgeon is so confident in his prosthesis that he often does bilateral keratoprostheses and has the clock running on both, simultaneously.

Most people who are monocular have adapted to that condition and can perform most visual tasks, except those few tasks that require good steriopsis. It seems ill advised to have the clock running on both eyes simultaneously, knowing that trauma could cause the loss of both prostheses, or that both prostheses could be infected or extruded at the same time. By doing only one eye at a time, until it is successful or has failed completely, we could prolong the useful vision for many years through what is now considered a temporary, albeit sometimes long lasting, restoration of vision, when it is performed sequentially in the two eyes.

Part Seven

Current Prostheses

Prostheses of several types are in use or under evaluation today, but all have complications. Use of the osteo-odonto-keratoprosthesis has spread from Italy to England, Germany, and the United states. Worst is using the Champaign cork prosthesis that he designed in Europe and Singh, in India, is using a Worst wheel rim design. Dohlman is using his Type I and II prostheses with the anterior and posterior plates along with a mandatory glaucoma drain and reservoir. The Seoul prosthesis, the Pintucci prosthesis and the Legeais prosthesis all have cores of PMMA and skirts of synthetic fiber and are among the most successful. There is also the Chirila prosthesis, a unique lamellar design, and the Caldwell prosthesis with a urethane lens and Gore-Tex® haptic. Each of these incorporates some of the improved features discussed, but each has design flaws. None have become uniformly successful as detailed below.

Osteo-odonto-keratoprosthesis Although Falcinelli claims almost complete success, others report failure of this prosthesis because of extrusion and infection. The Strampelli/Falcinelli prosthesis relies on the patient having good teeth and bone as well as adequate oral mucosa. Therefore, this prosthesis can not be used in some patients with Stevens-Johnson syndrome, ocular cicatricial pemphigoid and severe Sjogren's syndrome (dry eye, dry mouth, and arthritis) because they have bad dentition and poor quality oral mucosa. Patients who dip snuff or chew tobacco also have oral mucosa unsuitable for grafting.

Worst Champagne Cork Prosthesis Singh Prosthesis These prostheses are still in use, but suffer from problems with the stainless steel sutures. Because they have no biointegration, the tension on the sutures causes them to erode through the tissues leading to instability of the prosthesis and damage to the eye. Singh's reports of success are based on her criterion for success: When the patient does not return from distant parts of India for follow up, the prosthesis is assumed successful. This is probably unrealistic considering the transportation available and distances traveled by the patients and the fact that failure may prompt seeking another physician rather than returning to the unsuccessful one.

Dohlman Type-I and *II Prostheses* Dohlman reports success with his prosthesis now that he routinely uses a glaucoma reservoir and covers his prosthesis with a soft bandage contact lens. This prosthesis has no biointegration which may explain why there are still melting problems which he treats with Provera® eye drops. The high incidence of glaucoma is a definite problem with this prosthesis.

The Seoul Prosthesis The developers of the Seoul Prosthesis are claiming success with this prosthesis, but they have reported some delayed extrusion of the skirt due to depopulation of the fibrous tissue of the skirt.

Legeais Prosthesis Pouliquen has reported late failure of this prosthesis for the same reason as the Seoul prosthesis and it may be out of use.

Chirila Prosthesis The Chirila prosthesis has a unique design–an alloplastic tissue which is used in place of a lamellar corneal tissue graft. Because of the exposure of the alloplastic material and its failure to support an epithelium in the dry eye, it remains contraindicated in recurrent herpes simplex, atrophic corneas, and the advanced dry eye. All of these conditions are causes for failure of corneal transplants. Multiple transplant failure is a prime indication for keratoprosthesis surgery. There have been reports of success in other diseases.

Caldwell's "soft keratoprosthesis" This prosthesis depends on strips of a haptic material being incorporated into the sclera and bonding of the core or lens to the haptic material. He has reported failures with the bonding between optic and haptic and the scleral incorporation on the haptic material.

Part Eight

Design of a New Prosthesis

Analysis of the reports of the periodic conferences of the Keratoprosthesis Study Group indicates that many of the researchers now working in the field believe that the retention of a keratoprosthesis depends on a combination of mechanical and biological factors which must be considered in the design of a successful prosthesis.

Incorporation of many of the beneficial modifications learned from the past and through recent experimentation, while avoiding those which have not proved useful, could produce a successful keratoprosthesis. This prosthesis could have improved retention in the eye for an extended period of time.

The most notable of the factors to be considered are:

1. A properly sized and shaped biocolonizable skirt to obliterate the tissue to alloplastic interface through fibrovascular integration of the skirt material,
2. Permanent mechanical and chemical attachment of the skirt to the core to avoid failure from separation of the two,
3. An anterior flange on the core to prevent conjunctival overgrowth of the prosthesis core,
4. Biointegration between alloplastic material and tissue that obstructs the epithelial downgrowth that separates the skirt or core from the cornea and also creates glaucoma,
4. A cone shaped core to inhibit retroprosthetic membranes and to force the posterior corneal lamella against the skirt to prevent lamellar separation from the skirt,
5. The preparation of the implant site to receive the prosthesis, and.
6. The use of antibiotics, heparin, and steroids to prevent inflammation and subsequent membrane formation.

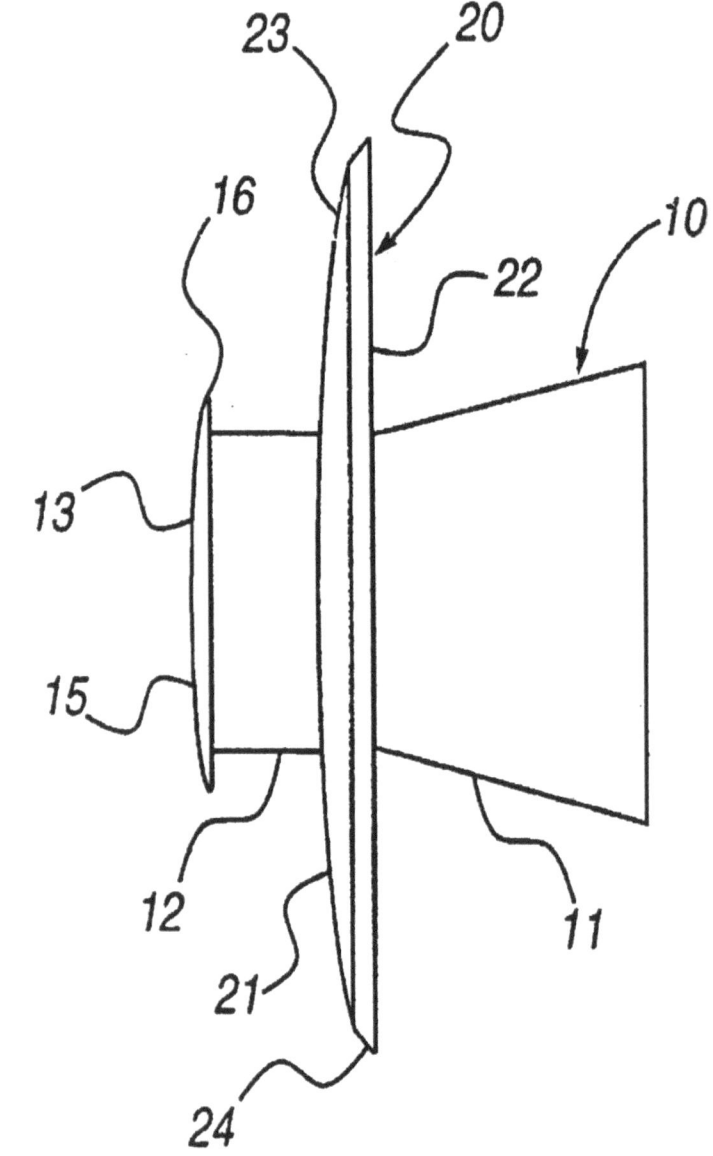

Figure 2. Keratoprosthesis of a new composite design. 10 = Polymethyl methacrylate (PMMA) core; 11 = conical portion; 12 = cylindrical portion;13 = optical portion; 15 = optical surface; 16 = anterior flange; 20 = fibrous skirt; 21 = convex anterior surface; 22 = concave posterior surface; 23 = radius of curvature 9.5 mm; 24 = beveled edge.

Part Nine

Animal Research

Ten prostheses were produced that incorporated the significant features which have been shown to enhance retention and promote visual success. A series of ten implantations in cat corneas was performed, using a surgical technique that has been developed over years of trials, in order to evaluate characteristics and procedures that would promote retention of the prosthesis.

This is a prospective, non-blinded study without a control procedure. There is no consensus of a successful prosthesis that could be available to the investigator to use as a control. The feline teeth and jaw bones are not suitable for the osteo-odonto-keratoprosthesis in cats. Other prostheses were not available for use in this research.

The cats were evaluated for time of extrusion or the full-term retention of the prosthesis. Clinical study of eyes was performed periodically during and after the retention or expulsion of the prosthesis. All eyes were examined histologically at the end of the study, including any eye which had extruded the prosthesis.

Materials and methods The prosthesis consisted of a PMMA optical core with a white Proplast® skirt that was joined by both mechanical forces and methyl cyanoacrylate adhesive. The central hole in the skirt was 4 mm in diameter to fit in the grove in the 5 mm core cylinder. Each prosthesis core was manufactured and joined to a commercially manufactured skirt in the ophthalmology laboratory.

The prosthesis core was cut from a cylindrical blank of intraocular-lens-grade PMMA using a contact lens lathe. The blank had been cut to 7 mm thickness from a rod 11 mm in diameter. The rod of polymerized PMMA, furnished by IOLAB Corporation (Claremont, California), had been removed from a tube in the molding machine at the end of a run of extrusion molding of intraocular lenses manufactured for human use. This material is compatible with intraocular use.

Each blank was lathe polished to a smooth cylinder 10 mm in diameter and end polished to a length of 6.5 mm. The blank was mounted in the chuck of a contact lens swing lathe. The lathe was used to make a smooth 60 Diopter curved surface on the exposed end of the blank. This surface was then polished to optical smoothness using contact lens techniques. The working piece was detached from the chuck and the opposite surface was then polished flat using a standard contact lens polishing machine.

Both polished surfaces were mounted in chucks for the lathe using the red wax commonly used for contact lens manufacture. The piece was then lathe-cut to a cylinder with a diameter of 6 mm throughout the entire length. Using diamond tipped tools, the anterior, or optically curved, end was undercut at the edge of the curved surface. This cut was made perpendicular to the cylinder axis, to create a core diameter of 5.0 mm extending for a distance of 1.5 mm from the undercut edge. This created a 0.5 mm overhang or flange at the anterior end of the core, the purpose of which was to prevent overgrowth of the conjunctiva and to promote smooth movement of the eyelid over the optical core. The lathe cut was extended further away from the anterior end to form a tapering cone with an anterior diameter of 5.0 mm that enlarged to 6.0 mm diameter at the posterior end. A 0.5 mm wide and 0.25 mm deep groove was cut into the cylinder core immediately anterior to the junction of the cylinder and cone parts, leaving 1 mm of 5.0 mm diameter cylinder core behind the anterior cap. The lathe cut surface was made as smooth as possible using cutting tools, but left optically opaque, rather than polished. This was done to minimize internal reflection from the core sides as recommended by Cardona. The core was then removed from the red clay mounting and both optical surfaces lightly polished using a standard contact lens polishing machine to smooth them before the skirt was mounted.

At this point the core was 6.0 mm long to provide for 2.5 to 3.0 mm posterior protrusion behind the cornea. (1 mm optical cap, 1 mm anterior core, 0.5 mm skirt groove, and 3.5 mm conical posterior core to allow 0.5 mm to 1.0mm posterior cornea lamella around the conical core.)

The skirts were made by Vitek, Inc. in Houston, Texas, manufacturer of Proplast®. Ten millimeters round disks were cut from sheets of 0.3 mm thick Proplast® using a 10 mm trephine. This thickness of Proplast® had been shown to have good biointegration with the cornea[23]. A 4.0 mm trephine was used to make a hole in the center of the disk to create a tight fit in the groove of the core. The outer edges of the disk were then manually shaved, using Xacto® blades, so that the outer edge was no more than 0.15 mm thick (half thickness) with a smooth taper to avoid pressure points against the cornea. The skirts were shaped to have an approximate posterior radius of curvature of 9.5 mm. (the central curvature of the cat cornea).

The core and skirt were assembled by hand in the ophthalmology laboratory using ophthalmic surgery instruments. Super glue was applied sparingly to the entire groove. The skirt was then worked over the anterior flange of the core and pulled posteriorly using non-toothed forceps until the skirt seated in the groove. The tight fit and glue seal attachment was designed to block epithelial downgrowth and prevent separation of the core and skirt.

After overnight drying under ultraviolet light, the prostheses were cleaned with alcohol and packaged for gas sterilization using ethylene gas. The sterile prosthesis was fully aerated before use.

Experimental animals The cat was chosen as the experimental animal for a number of reasons. Cats are very fastidious, adapt well to laboratory life, and require a minimum of care, making it relatively inexpensive to keep them for long periods of time. They live for many years making it possible to study long term retention of a prosthesis.

Moodie and others[62] found the central corneal curvature in the adult cat to be 39 D, compared to 45 D for humans. Using ultrasound biometry, Gilger[63] and colleagues determined that the ocular length of the cat eye to be 20.91 +/- 0.53 mm which is similar to the axial length of about 23 mm for humans. The central corneal thickness was also found by Gilger[64] and colleagues to be 578 +/- 64 microns by ultrasonic pachymetry. This is similar to the average of 540 microns for humans. According to Hayashi and co-workers[66], the cat cornea does have a Bowman's layer which is much thinner than Bowman's layer in the human eye. Bahn and colleagues[65] said that the regenerative capacity of the corneal endothelium in the cat, like that of the human, is limited and he concluded, "...this cooperative hardy animal is an excellent model in which to study many aspects of corneal transplantation that have direct application to the treatment of human corneal disease".

Other differences include the presence of a nictitating membrane, or third eyelid, and the tendency for aqueous humor of cats to clot on exposure to air. This also happens in rabbits and children, but not in the normal adult human. To overcome these differences, the nictitating membrane was surgically removed before the implantation and 0.1 ml of heparin was injected to the anterior chamber prior to exposing the aqueous humor to air.

The cat crystalline lens can be removed by phacoemulsification more easily than in dogs although the tough posterior capsule of the cat is prone to opacification if left intact.

Primates might have been a better model for corneal similarity, but were considered too expensive and too difficult to manage for the frequent examinations, just to overcome the minor discrepancies with the cat cornea.

Ten short-hair American cats of mixed breeds were acquired through the animal care services of the university. These cats were claimed, pre-euthanasia, from animal pounds outside of the Galveston area. The use of animals was approved and monitored by the Animal Care Committee of the University of Texas Medical Branch. The Code for Animal Care for Research, as adopted by the Association for Research in Vision and Ophthalmology, was rigidly observed throughout the research.

Each cat was tattooed in one ear for identification purposes and immunized for distemper, feline leukemia, and other common feline diseases. The cats were isolated in the animal care facility for 3 weeks prior to being transferred to the ophthalmology cat laboratory, where they remained isolated from other cats and other species throughout the experimental period.

The cats were fed Purina Cat Chow *ad libitum* and provided with fresh water daily. All cats were allowed to roam the cat laboratory for at least 1 hour per day and became tame to the investigators and caretakers.

A safe technique had been developed in this laboratory to anesthetize the cats with Halothane inhalation anesthesia which produced good levels of anesthesia with no loss of animal life.

Experimental procedures The cats each received a keratoprosthesis in one eye only. The Animal Care Committee specifically prohibited doing anything which would compromise or interfere with vision from the opposite eye at any time during the study and prohibited use of any animal with impaired vision in the non-operated eye.

The anesthesia technique used for surgery on cats had been developed in the ophthalmology laboratory with the assistance of a small-animal veterinarian who taught cat intubation to all of the involved investigators. The cats were given general endotracheal anesthesia with halothane, nitrous oxide, and oxygen, with cardiac monitoring to observe and adjust depth of anesthesia.

For anesthesia induction, the cat was placed in a Plexiglas® box that was large enough for the cat to stand comfortably. The tubing from the gas machine was connected to the box and the box was filled with a mixture of oxygen, nitrous oxide, and halothane. When the cat had reached an appropriate stage of anesthesia, the cat was removed from the box and intubated by direct laryngoscopy using a non-cuffed endotracheal tube. The lungs were checked by stethoscope to be sure the tube was correctly placed.

Anesthesia machine settings were adjusted to allow the cat to breathe spontaneously while maintaining an adequate level of anesthesia. Cardiac rate was monitored during anesthesia to determine that the anesthetic level was appropriate. When surgery was complete, the halothane and nitrous oxide were turned off and the cat was awakened on pure oxygen. The cat was placed in his or her cage and allowed to awaken fully.

All cats received a minimum of four surgical procedures in the course of implantation of a prosthesis. Two procedures were done to prepare the cat eye for the prostheses. In the third procedure the prosthesis was implanted and covered with conjunctiva. The conjunctiva was removed from the surface of the core in the fourth procedure. Additional procedures might be necessary in some cats to revise the conjunctival covering of the prosthesis.

Each cat was prepared for prosthesis surgery in the first procedure by removal of the nictitating membrane and suturing the conjunctival edges together at the base of the nictitating membrane. The crystalline lens was removed to avoid cataract formation during the evaluation period. Radial silk sutures were placed in the peripheral cornea to induce vascularization of the cornea.

In the actual procedure, the cat was anesthetized and placed in position for surgery on the eye. The hair around the eye was washed with Betadine® (Purdue Frederick Co. Stamford, Connecticut). The eye was draped with plastic drapes to exclude all hair from the field. A speculum was placed in the eye and the eye irrigated with Balanced Salt Solution® (Alcon Laboratories, Inc., Fort Worth, Texas).

The nictitating membrane was identified and clamped across the base using two hemostats, tip to tip. After sufficient time for hemostasis, the clamps were removed and the membrane was excised, without bleeding, along the hemostat crush marks. The incision line was then sutured closed with a running 6-0 chromic suture.

The crystalline lens was then extracted by phacoemulsification through a 3 mm limbal incision, leaving the posterior capsule intact. The incision was closed with one 10-0 suture. Twelve 9-0 silk sutures were placed radially in the peripheral cornea. These were placed in a clock dial manner spanning the 3 mm immediately within the limbus. Knots were left exposed and pulled to the central corneal end of the stitch to incite vascularization. Each cat received Tobradex ointment (Alcon) twice daily until the sutures were removed.

Two weeks after suture placement, the cat was again anesthetized and the corneal sutures were removed.

Within three weeks after suture removal, when the newly formed corneal vessels had emptied to become ghost vessels and all suture marks had healed, the cat's eye was ready for keratoprosthesis surgery.

During the actual procedure, the cat was anesthetized, prepared and draped for surgery as previously described. An eyelid speculum was placed in the eye that had been previously prepared to receive the prosthesis and the eye was irrigated with Balanced Salt Solution (Alcon).

The cornea was inspected for vascularization and the scar from the nictitating membrane was checked for healing. If the healing was complete, the conjunctiva was dissected from the limbus in a 360 degree peritomy. The conjunctiva was freed by blunt dissection from underlying Tenon's capsule as far out from the limbus as possible in all directions. Hemostasis was obtained with thermal cautery. All epithelium was scraped from the cornea and limbus using a #15 Bard-Parker blade. Removal of all epithelium was verified with fluorescein staining.

Using a #59 Beaver blade, a half thickness perpendicular incision, 12 mm long, was made along the temporal limbus at the edge of clear cornea. A lamellar dissector was used to separate the cornea into two layers creating a half depth corneal pocket starting from the bottom of this incision and extending across the entire cornea. A stab incision was made at the limbus into the anterior chamber away from the initial incision. Heparin, 0.1 milliliter, was injected into the anterior chamber.

The center of the cornea was located and marked. A 4 mm corneal trephine, centered on the mark, was used to make a hole completely through both layers of the cornea. The central 4 mm buttons were removed from both layers of the cornea.

The prosthesis was grasped with smooth forceps and introduced into the intralamellar pocket. The prosthesis was positioned so that the anterior core protruded through the anterior lamellar hole and the posterior lamellar hole was aligned with the posterior end of the core. Position of the skirt was checked and corrected as needed with a spatula. The anterior chamber was inflated with Balanced Salt Solution (Alcon) through the stab incision until the posterior core snapped through the posterior hole. Intraocular pressure was then adjusted by injecting or removing fluid through the stab incision.

The limbal incision was then sutured with a continuous 10-0 nylon suture. The conjunctiva was advanced and closed in a linear running fashion using 6-0 chromic suture to approximate the edges and to cover the cornea and prosthesis completely with conjunctiva. Tobradex ointment and drops (Alcon) were placed in the eye. The speculum and drapes were removed and the cat was allowed to awaken.

Each cat was examined daily without anesthesia to determine whether the conjunctival flap was in place and flat against the cornea and prosthesis and free of inflammation or purulent discharge. Cats were observed for four to six weeks before the core was exposed. The behavior of the cat and the appearance of the eyelids for signs of rubbing were watched as indications of pain in the eye. Each cat received Tobradex Ointment (Alcon) once daily until the core was exposed.

Cores were exposed once conjunctival edema and any other inflammation had subsided. The cat was anesthetized, positioned, and draped for eye surgery. A speculum was placed in the eye and the conjunctiva was irrigated with Balanced Salt Solution® (Alcon). The core was easily located by the protrusion in the conjunctival flap. The conjunctiva was elevated over the core and incised, being careful not to scratch the core. The incision was extended to open a round hole slightly smaller than the anterior core. This opening was forced over the flange of the anterior core and as far posteriorly as possible. Tobradex drops were placed into the eye and the cat was allowed to awaken.

Tobradex ointment (Alcon) was placed in each operated eye twice each day for five days after exposure of the core or repair of the conjunctiva. Thereafter, each eye received Prednisilone Acetate 1% eye drops, (Alcon) daily for the duration of the study.

If the conjunctiva retracted from the core or other gaps in conjunctival coverage of the cornea occurred, the cat was anesthetized, prepared with Betadine® solution and draped. A speculum was placed in the eye for exposure. The retracted conjunctiva around the opening was freed from underlying tissue, advanced to cover the cornea, and sutured with 6-0 chromic sutures to close the gap and bring the conjunctiva tightly around the prosthesis core.

Evaluation procedures Each eye was examined daily for evidence of retraction of the conjunctiva away from the core, holes in the conjunctiva, signs of inflammation, purulent discharge, or change in the light reflex through the prosthesis. Eyes were examined with a portable slit lamp (Kowa) and a small pupil indirect ophthalmoscope (Keeler) each week for signs of retroprosthetic membranes or retinal detachment and checked at that time by gentle finger pressure on the eyeball for evidence of elevated intraocular pressure.

Results Keratoprostheses were placed in one eye in each of ten cats. Nine of the implants were retained for the duration of the study. The prostheses were well accepted by the corneas and were well centered within the limbus. There was a rapid decrease of swelling and inflammation in the conjunctival flap. Two cats developed retraction of the conjunctiva from the core requiring repair, one each at the fourth and eighth weeks. Both repairs were successful in obtaining conjunctival coverage of the cornea for the duration of the study.

The conjunctiva formed a tight seal with the optical core and did not grow across the optical portion. The conjunctival flaps thinned to permit easy visualization of the optical core and skirt in the cornea (Figures 3, 4).

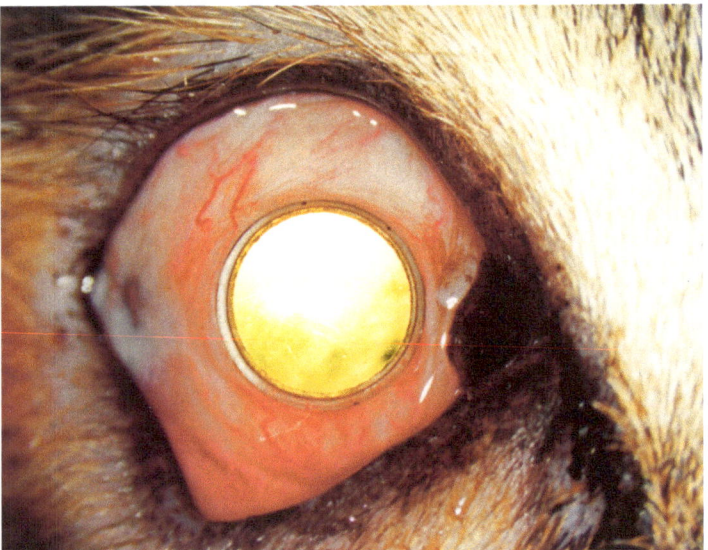

Figure 3 Frontal view, right eye, cat with prosthesis, six months after implantation. Eye is not inflamed. Prosthesis is in good position with flange visible above conjunctiva. Good tapetal reflex. (6X)

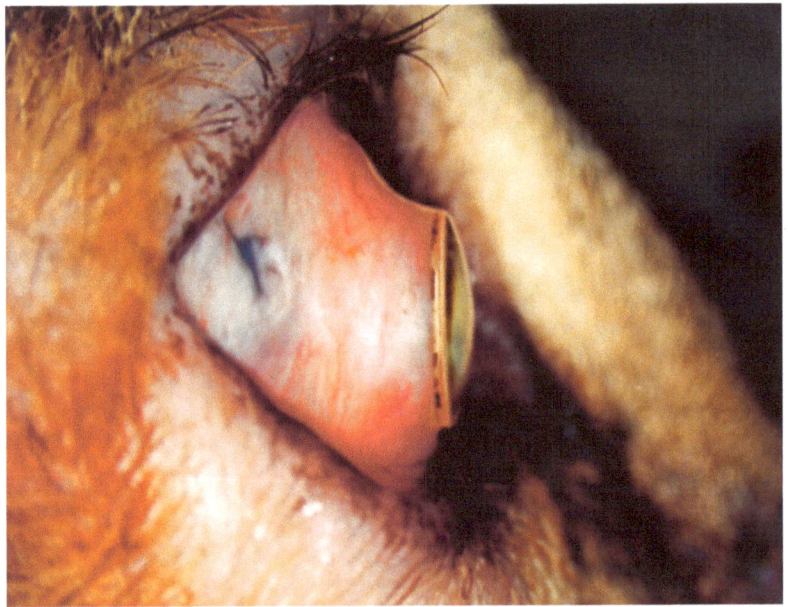

Figure 4 Same eye as figure 3. Lateral view, six months after implantation. Non-inflamed conjunctiva surrounding prosthesis core up to anterior flange. (6X)

One prosthesis was extruded at week eight because of retraction of a previously undetected retroprosthesis membrane. The membrane was substantial enough to prevent loss of intraocular contents. A retroprosthetic membrane was found in one other eye at week eleven and was immediately removed surgically. The membrane did not recur.

There were no infections, either conjunctival or intraocular. Intraocular pressure remained low in all cats as evidenced by softness to tactile pressure. There was no erosion of the skirt through the conjunctiva or peripheral gaps in the conjunctival covering. The cats appeared comfortable throughout the post operative period without signs of eye rubbing or eyelid ptosis to indicate pain, uveitis or ocular irritation, (Figure 5). The cats were examined using the indirect ophthalmoscope every week. The view became hazy in some cats due to opacification of the lens capsule, but no retinal detachments occurred. The only changes to the tapetal light reflex were thought to be caused by lens capsule opacification. The Nd/YAG laser was not available in the laboratory to open these capsules.

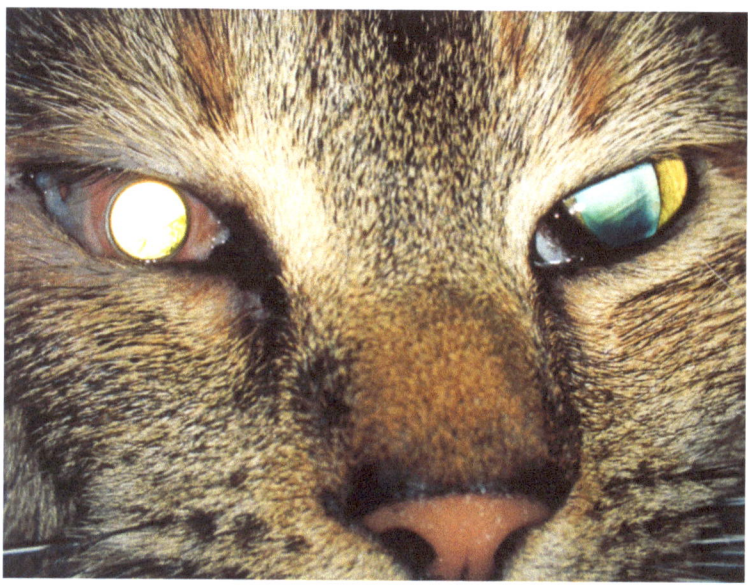

Figure 5 Frontal view of a cat with a keratoprosthesis in the right eye. Note the lack of ptosis or loss of eyelid hair that would indicate irritation, pain, or photophobia caused by the prosthesis.

The Animal Care Committee prohibited obstruction of the non operated eye at any time. The cats did not show the sideways movements into the field of vision usually seen with animals that are blind in one eye when they were allowed to move about the laboratory. The cats were not trained for visual acuity measurement.

The study was terminated at 6 months after implantation due to a change in academic institution of the principle investigator and the cessation of grant funding which was linked to the institution where the work was done.

The cats were sacrificed (university policy) and the eyes with implants were enucleated and fixed in formalin. In all nine eyes that retained a prosthesis, the implant was firmly fixed in the cornea. The PMMA cores of the prostheses were dissected from the corneas and the eyes were processed for histopathological study, including fixation in formalin, clearing with xylene, embedding in paraffin, microtome sectioning (at 5 μm) and staining with hematoxylin and eosin and with periodic acid Schiff (PAS) stains.

Gross examination of the formalin fixed eyes showed that the Proplast® was firmly attached to the cornea, the anterior chambers were well formed, and there were no retinal detachments (Figure 6). The cores had to be removed before sectioning and were all found to be firmly attached to the skirts.

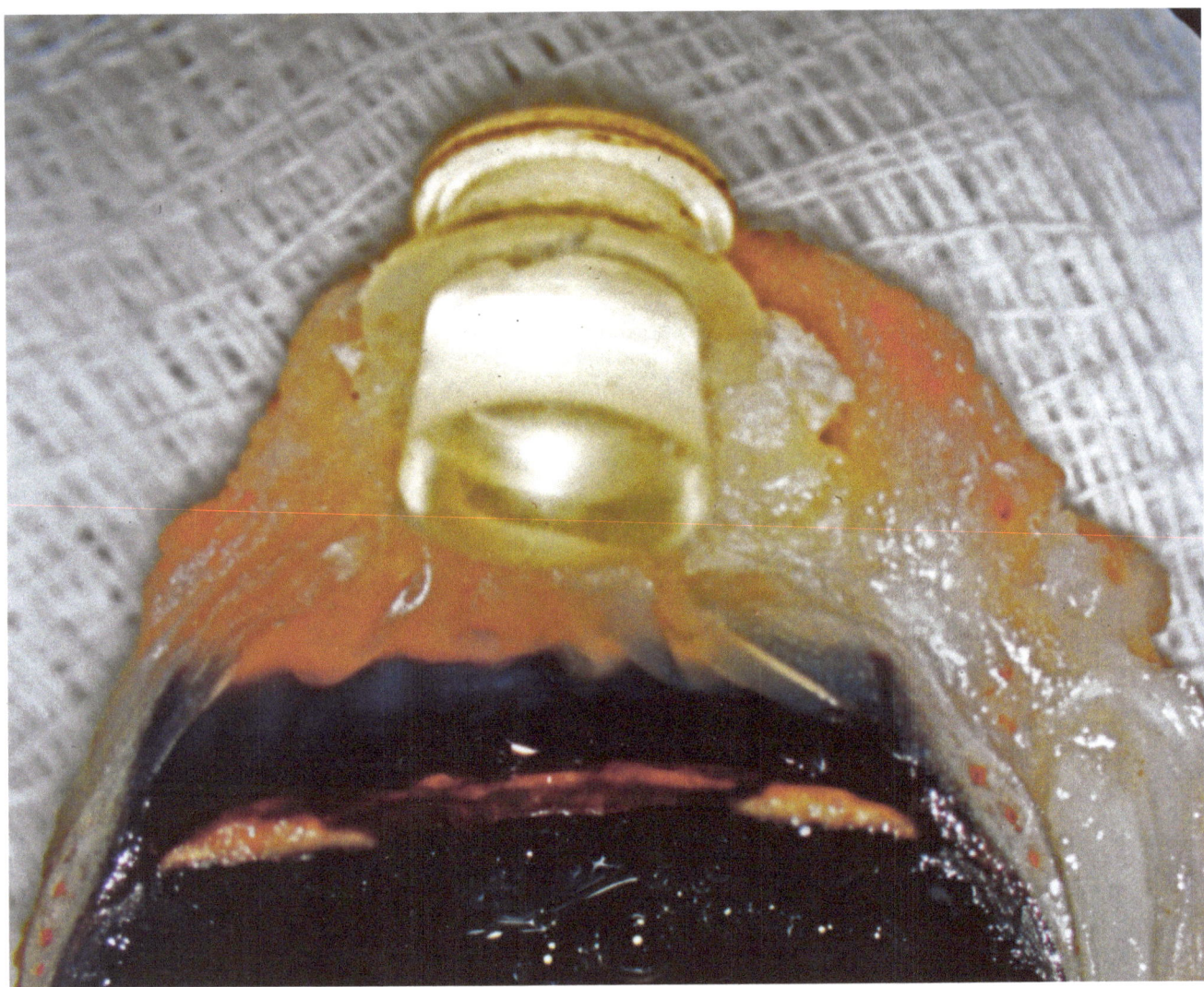

Figure 6 Section of cat eye with prosthesis in place. The prosthesis has been dissected from the other half of the cornea to separate the two halves of the eye. The prosthesis is in good position without a retroprosthesis membrane on the core. The iris is well back from the posterior cornea with open angle structures.

On microscopic examination of serial sections of the nine eyes that retained the prosthesis, fibrovascular incorporation of the entire Proplast® skirt was found (Figure 7). No evidence of retroprosthetic membrane formation was seen in any of these nine corneas, including the one in which the membrane was removed in week eleven. There was good approximation of the conjunctiva to the cornea with no epithelial downgrowth between the conjunctiva and cornea, or between the cornea and prosthesis core or skirt. The interstices of the Proplast® were filled with blood vessels. The PAS stained sections showed fibrous tissue throughout the skirt material. (Figure 8).

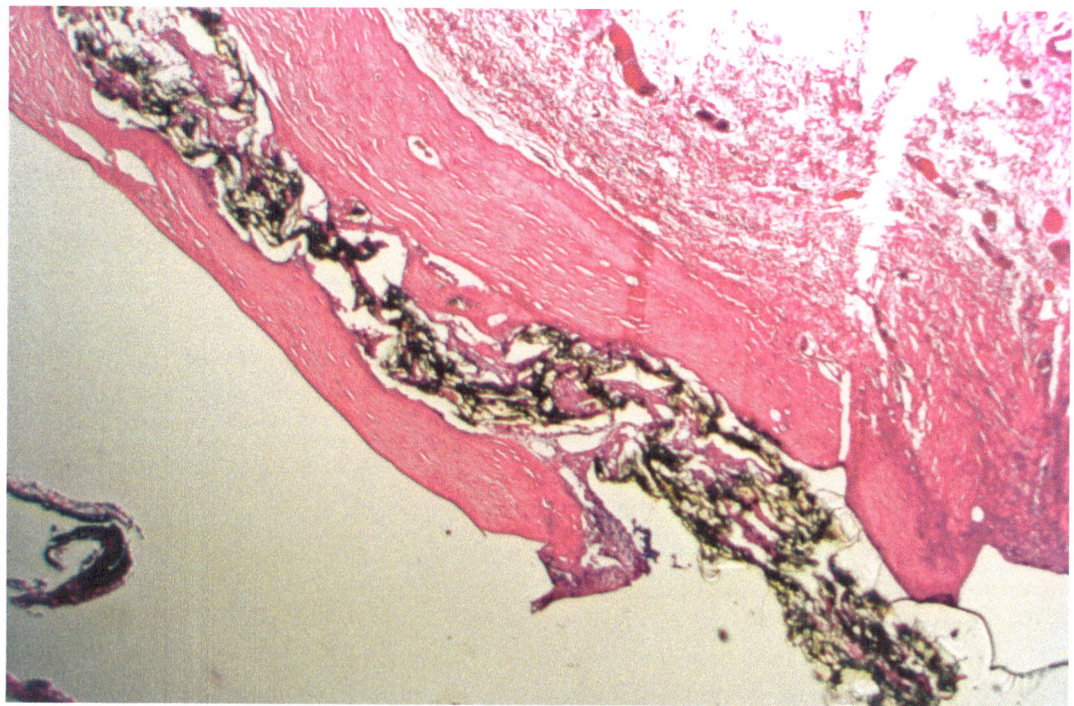

Figure 7 Section of the cornea containing the Proplast® skirt material (Black).Fibrous tissue and blood vessels within the interstices of the Proplast®. Note absence of inflammatory response, no epithelium between the Proplast® and the cornea, and iris is behind the cornea, but not adherent, due to processing artifact. (PAS, X50)

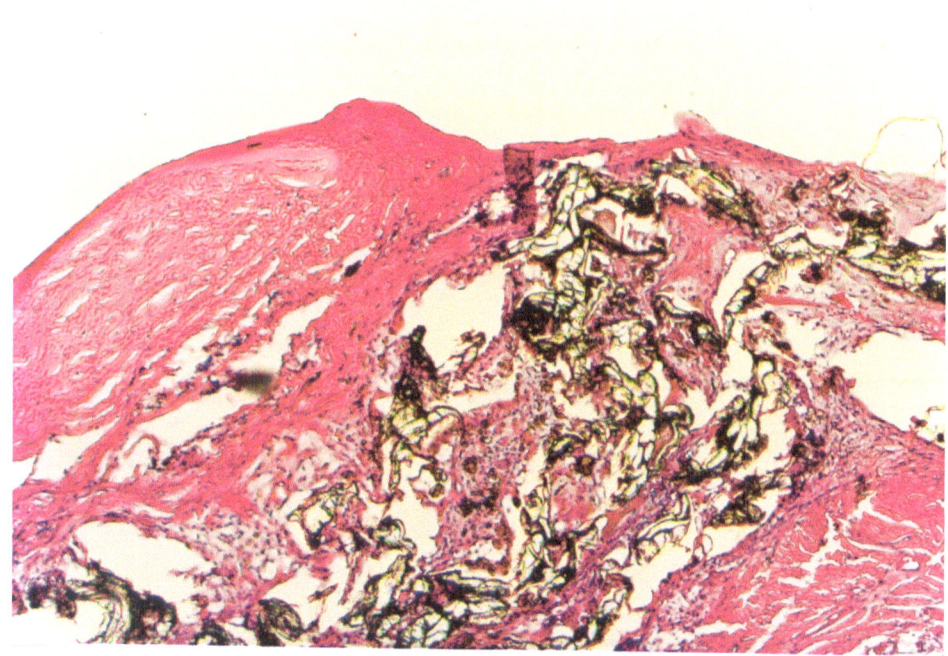

Figure 8 Section of Cornea containing Proplast with fibrous tissue and blood vessels within the Proplast®. Conjunctiva on the surface of the cornea with thickening at the edge of the cornea where the prosthesis core was attached. No epithelial downgrowth or inflammatory cells in the corneal stroma (PAS, X125)

Examination of the skirt of the prosthesis that had been extruded revealed patches of Proplast® which were free of fibrovascular invasion. The eye that had expelled the implant had a retroprosthetic membrane spanning the corneal opening. The membrane prevented collapse of the anterior chamber. There was no evidence of epithelial downgrowth.

Discussion The prosthesis described in this paper appears to have promise for long term retention in the cornea. It incorporates many of the beneficial features and overcomes many of the difficulties posed by previous keratoprostheses.

The conjunctiva did not grow past the anterior flange of the core, but formed a tight seal around the core. (Figure 6) This indicates that the elevated flange is effective in preventing this complication. The tight seal should prevent epithelial collagenase from reaching the corneal stroma around the core.

The Proplast skirt provided good biointegration between the cornea and the prosthesis. The presence of vessels in the Proplast® skirt should prevent collagenolytic activity in the surrounding cornea.

The tight seal between the core and the skirt was effective in blocking any epithelial downgrowth along the core. Downgrowth around the skirt did not occur which was probably because of the rapid biointegration of the skirt from the previously vascularized cornea. This preparatory vascularization step is critical to the incorporation of the prosthesis into a normal cornea. Many eyes requiring a prosthesis are already vascularized from the disease process, but some may have segmental vascularization and will need procedures to vascularize the cornea completely prior to implantation.

The posterior lamella of the cornea was well approximated to the posterior side of the skirt. Whether this is because of the conical shape of the core or because of early biointegration was not determined. This may have played a role in the low number of retroprosthetic membranes. The use of steroids throughout the post implant period may also have contributed to the lack of membrane formation.

Unfortunately, the early termination of this study did not allow for determination of the total length of time that this prosthesis could be maintained in the cornea. In previous experiments, prosthesis extrusion occurred between 2 weeks and 3 months after implantation when it occurred. The remaining prostheses were retained for more than a year. Because the prostheses that were in place at the end of this study were well anchored and free of complications at 6 months after implantation, it is probable that the prostheses could have been retained for a much longer period. One cat from a previous study retained a prosthesis with a cylindrical core, no anterior flange, and a 9 mm Proplast® skirt for 9 years, until an infection caused erosion around the core with expulsion of the prosthesis. Three other cats have retained a prior model of Proplast® skirt prosthesis for over four years.

The nature of keratoprosthesis research makes it difficult to compare these results with others. Most keratoprosthesis research, which is conducted outside the United States, is done directly in human subjects. The few animal studies that have been done are often not published, but serve only to satisfy the investigator that the prosthesis can be used in human subjects. Many studies are presented at meetings but not published

Animals do not report changes in the feel of the eye or changes in vision and must be examined frequently, so comparison of results of animal studies with investigations in human subjects, who are very aware of the feel of the prosthesis and subtle changes in vision or appearance of the prosthesis, is not appropriate. Early detection with corrective intervention is more difficult in animals causing poorer results. However, if the results in animals are better than in the human subjects, as they are in this study, the new prosthesis has promise.

The significant modifications in the design and use of this prosthesis give it several advantages over previous prostheses. They are as follows:

1. The small, slightly elevated, anterior flange prevents conjunctiva from growing across the core and allows the eyelid to move more easily over the prosthesis core.
2. The combined mechanical and adhesive attachment of the skirt to the core prevents mechanical separation of the core and skirt and prevents the growth of epithelium into the space between the core and skirt.
3. The conical shape of the posterior core forces the posterior corneal lamella against the skirt and also increases the visual field size
4. The large size of the skirt and material from which it is manufactured (stiff, but not hard, biocolonizable material) act to disperse the forces impinging upon the prosthesis onto to a broad area of the cornea.
5. The intralamellar placement of the skirt in a suitably vascularized cornea produces strong, rapid biointegration.
6. The prior vascularization of the cornea ensures a rich vascular bed from which the fibrovascular tissue can migrate from all directions to incorporate the entire skirt within days after implantation.
7. The small percentage of eyes that develop retroprosthesis membranes was unusual. It is not clear if this advantage is related to the design of the core (flared posteriorly), the use of heparin during implantation to prevent clotting of the aqueous on the core, or the control of infection and inflammation with steroids and antibiotics, or all of these. Worst, who used conical cores, has reported similar low rates of membrane formation.

Limitations of this Keratoprosthesis still exist. Proplast® is no longer available because the manufacturer is no longer in business and no other company is making this product. As a result, a substitute material must be found from which to manufacture the keratoprosthesis skirt. Pintucci showed that Dacron® felt works well as a material for a keratoprosthesis skirt. It is well incorporated into the cornea. This material could be substituted for the Proplast®. Dacron® felt is porous, wettable, biocolonizable, and suitably rigid, yet soft enough to avoid pressure necrosis. It has been used for many years in vascular grafts and in Pintucci's keratoprosthesis.

Pintucci's prosthesis differs from the prosthesis described in this paper in that Pintucci's prosthesis uses a cylindrical core. There is no anterior flange, posterior taper to the core diameter, or groove in which the skirt can seat, all of which would be advantageous. Pintucci's design uses a less-secure attachment of the core to the skirt compared to the prosthesis described in this paper.

The Future of this Keratoprosthesis is now in question. Retention in the cornea of 9 of the 10 keratoprostheses in an animal eye for the duration of the study is a significant step in development of a keratoprosthesis that can be retained in human eyes for a long time. This study demonstrated that attention to both mechanical forces on the prosthesis and the promotion of biointegration of the prosthesis facilitates long-term retention of a keratoprosthesis. The author believes that this design, using a Dacron® felt skirt is now ready for human trials.

Present rules of the U.S. Food and Drug Administration[66] require that all investigations of devices in human subjects must be conducted under the auspices of a corporation with adequate corporate liability insurance. The ideal manufacturer of this device would be a company that is now engaged in the manufacture of intraocular lenses by pressure molding or lathe cutting and is also active in the distribution of other ophthalmic products throughout the world. . Some research in this country is considered grandfathered if the investigator was implanting prostheses prior to enactment of device regulations.

The use of keratoprostheses in the United States is limited by the aggressive use of donor tissue and the reluctance of most cornea surgeons to do keratoprosthesis surgery. There are many parts of the world where corneal blindness is common and transplant tissue is not available. Vitamin A deficiency is rampant in the Middle East and causes minor corneal injury to progress to total corneal blindness. In India, Hindu people believe in reincarnation so eye donors are scarce while corneal blindness is common. This device could restore vision to thousands or even millions of people throughout the world. The implantation procedure is simple and could easily be taught to ophthalmologists in the third world.

The manufacture of the optical cores and the skirts could be easily adapted to mass production by injection molding of the cores and assembly line methods of cutting and shaping of medical grade Dacron® felt. The assembling and attaching the two parts is very simple, less skill demanding than gluing micro cutting needles onto 10-0 nylon suture.

Acknowledgments

The author would like to acknowledge the assistance of Charles Homsy, MD, Ph.D. of Baylor College of Medicine and Vitek, Inc. and thank them for their assistance with the Proplast® skirt material and the manufacture and donation of the skirts for these prostheses.

The author also would like to thank the IOLAB Corporation, Claremont, California for supplying the ophthalmic grade polymethyl methacrylate rods which were used for the manufacture of the cores.

This work could not have been completed without the generous funding from the Walls Medical Research Foundation and the kind encouragement and dedication of Dr. Ned Dudney, Research director, and Mr. Carmage Walls, President, of the Walls Research Foundation.

The author would like to acknowledge the able assistance of Shirley, Kathy, and Young, my research assistants who cared for the cats, assisted at surgery and assisted with and performed the follow up examinations. Young Chung was very adept at the use of the swing lathe to manufacture the prosthesis cores once we designed and produced them together.

All of the investigators and technicians were generously trained in the anesthesia of cats by the late Patrick Ross Davidson, DVM.

Thanks are due to Dr. Claes Dohlman of Massachusetts Eye and Ear Infirmary and Dr S. Pintucci of Rome, Italy, for their frank discussions with me about their prostheses at various meetings of the Keratoprosthesis Study Group.

This work was performed at the Department of Ophthalmology of the University of Texas Medical Branch in Galveston Texas.

The author holds the U.S. Patent Number 5,489,301 issued February 6, 1996, titled Cornea Prosthesis.

References

1. Parel JM. 200 years of KPro: Pellier de Quengsy and the artificial Cornea. An. Inst Barraquer, (Barc) 1999;28 (Suppl.) 33-41. (Entire original article by De Quengsy reprinted in French.)

2. Cardona H. Keratoprosthesis—acrylic optical cylinder with supporting intralamellar plastic artificial disc. Am J Ophthalmol. 1962;88: 190-204.

3. Dimmer F. Zwei Falle fon Celluloidplatten de Hornhaut. Klin Monatsbl Augenheilkd. 1891;29:104-105.

4. Gyorffy J. Acrylic corneal implant in keratoplasty. Am J Ophthalmol. 1951; 34:757-758.

5. Dorzee M. Keratoprosthese Acrylic. Bull Soc Belge Ohthalmol. 1955; 108:582.

6. Stone W Jr. Study of patency of openings in corneas anterior to intralamellar plastic artificial disc. Am J Ophthalmol. 1955:39(2): 185-196.

7. Barraquer J. Early Experience and present views on Keratoprosthesis. An Inst Barraquer (Barc) 2001;30:33.

8. Binder H, Binder R. Experiments on Plexiglas corneal implants. Am J Ophthalmol. 1956; 41:793-797.

9. Cardona H. Plastic Keratoprostheses—a description of the plastic material and comparative histologic study of recipient corneas. Am J Ophthalmol.1964;58:247-252.

10. Choyce DP. Management of endothelial corneal dystrophy with acrylic corneal inlays. Brit J Ophthalmol. 1965; 3:307-311.

11. Roper-Hall MJ. How I became involved with keratoprosthesis. An Inst Barraquer (Barc). 2001;30:27-28.

12. Girard LJ, Moore CD, Soper JW, O'Bannon W. Prosthetosclero Keratoplasty—implantation of a keratoprosthesis using full thickness onlay sclera and sliding conjunctival flap. Trans Am Acad Ophthalmol Otolaryngol. 1969;73:936-961.

13. Girard LJ. Girard keratoprosthesis with flexible skirt: 28 years experience. Refractive Corneal Surg. 1993; 9:194-195.

14. Cardona H. Keratoprosthesis: acrylic optical cylinder with supporting intralamellar plate. Am J Ophthalmol. 1962;54; 284-294.

15. Cardona H, Castroviejo R, DeVoe AG. Techniques of prosthokeratoplasty: Further evaluation of results with the Cardona keratoprosthesis. Exc Med Int. 1966;146;837-847.

16. Dohlman CH, Schneider HA, Doane MG. Prosthokeratoplasty. Am J Ophthalmol. 1974; 77:694-700.

17. Dohlman CH. Biology of complications following keratoprosthesis. Cornea. 1983;2:175-179.

18. Strampelli B. Keratoprosthesis with osteodontal tissue. Am J Ophthalmol. 1963;89:1029-1039.

19. Falcinelli G, Barogi G, Taloni M, Falcinelli G: Osteoodontokeratoprosthesis: Present Experience and Future Prospects. Refractive Corneal Surg. 1993;9:193-194.

20. Polack FM, Heimke G. Ceramic Keratoprostheses. Ophthalmology. 1980; 87:693-698.

21. Kozarsky AM, Knight SH, Waring GO III. Clinical results with a ceramic keratoprosthesis placed through the eyelid. Ophthalmol. 1987;2:197-201.

22. Pintucci S, Pintucci F: New kind of keratoprosthesis. In: Pizzoferrato A, Marchetti P, Ravaglio A, Lee A, eds. Advances in Biomaterials, Vol 7, Elsevier Science Publishers B.V. 1987;321-324.

23. Barber JC, Feaster FT, Priour DJ. The acceptance of a vitreous carbon alloplastic material, Proplast®, into the rabbit eye. Invest Ophthalmol Vis Sci. 1980;19:182-190.

24. Barber JC. Keratoprosthesis: Past and present. Int Ophthalmol Clin. 1988; 28(2):103-109.

25. Legeais JM, Renard G, Rossi C, Salvoldelli M, DiHermies F Pouliguen Y. Keratoprosthesis: A comparative study of three different microporous polymer and first application in human eyes. Invest Ophthalmol Vis Sci. 1991;32(4):778.

26. Legeais JM Renard G, Pouliquen Y. Novel biocolonizable intrastromal keratoprosthesis: First year study in human. Invest Ophthalmol Vis Sci. 1993; 34:(Suppl):1367.

27. Lacombe E: Biocolonization: Early successes and late disillusions. An Inst Barraquer (Barc). 2002; 31:150-151.

28. Pintucci S, Pintucci F, Caiazza S. The Dacron felt colonizable keratoprosthesis. Refract Corneal Surg. 1993; 9:196-197.

29. Pintucci S, Pintucci F, Cecconi M, Caiazza S. The Pintucci's Dacron Tissue KP: How we improved the technique of implanting the KP in dry eyes and in eyes with sufficient tear secretion. Ann Inst Barraquer (Barc). 1999;28:(Suppl.): 51-56.

30. Worst JGF. 23 years of keratoprosthesis Research: Present state of the art. Refract Corneal Surg. 1993: 9:188-189.

31. van Andel P, Worst J, Singh I. Results of champagne cork Keratoprostheses in 127 Corneal Blind Eyes. An Inst Barraquer (Barc). 1993; 9:189-190.

32. Singh IR. Paralimbal scleral window. Ann Inst Barraquer (Barc). 2001;30:91-93.

33. Dohlman CH. Keratoprosthesis: Dohlman—Doane Types I and II; Brief description of operative procedure and postoperative regimen. Boston 1994.

34. Kim MK, Lee JL, Wee WR, and Lee JH. Comparative experiments for in vivo fibroplasia and biological stability for four porous polymers intended for use in the Seoul-type keratoprosthesis. Brit J of Ophthalmol. 2002; 86:809-814.

35. Chirila TV. Artificial cornea with a porous polymeric skirt. Trends Polym Sci. 1997; 5:(11):346-8.

36. Caldwell DR, The soft keratoprosthesis. Trans Am Ophthalmol Soc. 1997;95:751-802.

37. Trinkaus-Randall V, Banwatt RM, Wu XY, Liebositz HM, Franzblau C. Effect of pretreating porous webs on stromal fibroplasia in vivo. J Biomed Mater Res. 1994;28:195-202.

38. Castroviejo R, Cardona H, DeVoe AG. Present status of prostho-keratoplasty. Am J Ophthalmol. 1967; 64:228-233.

39. Turss R, Friend J, Dohlman CH. Effect of corneal fluid barrier on nutrition of the epithelium. Exp Eye Res. 1970;9:254.

40. Thoft RA, Friend J, Dohlman CH. Corneal Glucose Flux. Its response to anterior chamber blockade and endothelial damage. Arch Ophthalmol. 1971;86:685-691.

41. Slansky HH, Gnadinger MC, Itoi M, Dohlman CH. Collagenase in corneal ulceration. Arch Ophthalmol. 1969; 82:108-111.

42. Berman M, Kerza-Kwiatecki AP, Davison PF. Characterization of human corneal collagenase. Exp Eye Res. 1973;11: 255.

43. Berman MB, Barber JC, Talamo RC, Langley CE. Corneal ulceration and the serum antiproteases: I Alpha-1-antitrypsin. Invest Ophthalmol. 1973; 12:759-770.

44. Dohlman CH, Carroll JM, Ahmed B, Refojo ME. Replacement of the corneal epithelium with a contact lens (Artificial Epithelium). Trans Am Acad Ophthalmol Otolaryngol. 1969 May-June;73 (3): 482-493.

45. Newsome NA Gross J. Prevention by medroxyprogesterone of perforation in the alkali-burned rabbit cornea: Inhibition of collagenolytic activity. Invest Ophthalmol Vis Sci. 1977;16:21-31.

46. Lieberman J. Digestion of antitrypsin-deficient lung by leukoproteases in pulmonary emphysema and proteolysis. Mittman C, Ed. New York, 1972, Academic Press.

47. Stock EL, Aronson SB. Corneal Immune Globulin Distribution. Ann Ophthalmol. 1970 (Sep); 84(3):355-359.

48. Berman M. Regulation of corneal fibroblast MMP-1 secretion by plasmin. Cornea. 1993(Sep); 12(5):420-432.

49. Bath P, Mucosa RC, Cox K. Nd:YAG laser discission of retroprosthetic membrane: A preliminary report. Cornea. 1983; 2:225-228.

50. Ferry AP, Gordon BL. Epithelialization of the anterior chamber: A complication of prosthokeratoplasty. Arch Ophthalmol. 1974;91: 281-284.

51. Hille K, Landau H, Ruprecht KW. The Ahmed glaucoma valve in secondary glaucoma in osteo-odonto-keratoprosthesis. Ann Inst Barraquer (Barc). 2001; 30:139-141.

52. Hille K, Landau H, Ruprecht KW. Influence of the diameter of the PMMA cylinder on visual field in Osteo-odonto-keratoprosthesis. An Inst Barraquer (Barc). 201; 30:193-195.

53. Cardona H. Keratoprosthesis: Elimination of light reflection from the walls of the optical cylinder. Int Ophthalmol Clinics. 1966; 6(1):111-118.

54. Hull CC, Liu CSC, Sciscio A. Design of the osteo-odonto-keratoprosthesis optic: Improving the field of vision. An Inst Barraquer (Barc). 2001; 30:197-198.

55. Nio YK, Jansonius NM, Geraghty E, Norrby S, Kooijman AC. Effect of intraocular lens implantation on visual acuity, contrast sensitivity, and depth of focus. Cataract Refract Surg. 2003 Nov; 29(11):2073-81.

56. Barber J: Modifications of Keratoprosthesis to improve retention. Refrativ Corneal Surgery. 1993;9:200-201.

57. Castroviejo R, Cardona H, de Voe A. Symposium:keratoprosthesis, history, techniques, and indications. Trans Am Acad Ophthalmol Otolaryngol. 1977;83:249-251.

58. Temprano J. Keratoprosthesis with tibial autograft. Refract Corneal Surg. 1993;9:192-193.

59. Legeais JM, Renard G, Parel JM, Pouliguen Y. Expanded Polytetrafluoro-ethylene for keratoprosthesis skirt:Transparency and biocompatibility. Refract Corneal Surg. 1993;9:204-205.

60. Aquavella J, Bath P, Buxton G Polack F et al.. Keratoprosthesis Conference: roundtable discussion. Cornea. 1983; 2:229-236.

61. Polack FM, Heimke G. Ceramic Keratoprosthesis, long-term follow-up. An Inst Barraquer (Barc). 2001; 30:43-46.

62. Moodie KL, Hashizume N, Houston DL, Hoopes PJ, Demidenko E, Trembly BS, Davidson MG. Postnatal development of corneal curvature and thickness in the cat. Vet Ophthalmol. 2001;4:267-72.

63. Gilger BC, Davidson MG, Howard PB. Keratometry, ultrasonic biometry, and prediction of intraocular lens power in the feline eye. Am J Vet Res. 1998;59:131-4.

64. Gilger BC, Wright JC, Witley RD, McLaughlin SA. Corneal thickness measured by ultrasonic pachometry in cats. Am J Vet Res. 1993;54:228-30.

65. Bahn CF, Meyer RF, MacCallum DK, Lillie JH, Lovett EJ, Sugar A, Martonyi CL, Penetrating keratoplasty in the cat. A clinically applicable model. Ophthalmology, 1982;89:687-99.

66. Hayashi S, Osawa T, Tohyama K. Comparative observations on corneas, with special reference to Bowman's layer and Descemet's Membrane in mammals and amphibians. J Morphol, 2002;254:247-58.

67. Medical Devises. in FDA Information Sheets. U.S. Food and Drug Admin. 1998(Sep); 62-72.